# ESSENTIALS ~~OF~~
# EMERGENC~~Y~~ ~~MANAG~~EMENT
## Including the All-~~Hazards Ap~~roach

Brian J. Gallant

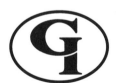

GOVERNMENT INSTITUTES

AN IMPRINT OF

THE SCARECROW PRESS, INC.

*Lanham, Maryland • Toronto • Plymouth, UK*

*2008*

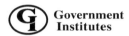 **Government Institutes**

Published in the United States of America
by Government Institutes, an imprint of The Scarecrow Press, Inc.
A wholly owned subsidiary of
The Rowman & Littlefield Publishing Group, Inc.
4501 Forbes Boulevard, Suite 200
Lanham, Maryland 20706
http://www.govinstpress.com/

Estover Road
Plymouth PL6 7PY
United Kingdom

British Library Cataloguing in Publication Information Available

**Library of Congress Cataloging-in-Publication Data**

Gallant, Brian.
  Essentials in emergency management : including the all-hazards approach /
Brian J. Gallant.
    p. cm.
  Includes index.
  ISBN-13: 978-0-86587-632-3 (pbk. : alk. paper)
  ISBN-10: 0-86587-632-0 (pbk. : alk. paper)
  1. Emergency management. I. Title.
  HV551.2.G35 2008
  363.34—dc22                                                2007051074

# Contents

*Contents*

# Figures and Tables

## Figures

## Tables

# Preface

THIS BOOK PROVIDES actionable information and ideas for new and existing emergency managers from various divisions, including homeland security and terrorism professionals; students in emergency management and homeland security programs; students studying environmental health and safety; firefighters and officers; police officials and law enforcement officers; local and city officials; consultants; disaster interruption managers; the media; and volunteers, their leaders, and agency supervisors (CERT, Red Cross, Salvation Army, and others); and anyone who deals with emergencies, disasters, and terrorism.

Whether paid or volunteer, emergency managers are overworked and under-appreciated. They are expected to be experts in a variety of subject areas, especially during the disaster phase of their job. While there are so many emergency management issues to deal with in this day and age that no text can be all-encompassing, the book outlines the various roles and responsibilities that emergency managers have in today's world and cover many of the major issues that an emergency manager will encounter, such as the natural hazards that they face every day and the technological hazards and terrorism issues that threaten our communities.

*Essentials in Emergency Management* discusses the Incident Command System (ICS) and the new presidential directive dealing with the National Incident Management Systems (NIMS). This book also discusses the new emergency management concept called the all-hazards approach, which is used by most communities, the states, and the federal government, and includes a description of the difference between it and the former Civil Defense of old. Also covered are issues such as managing volunteers, dealing with pets in disaster situations, and what the rest of the world is doing with respect to emergency management.

Finally, the appendices provide the reader with helpful reference materials, checklists, and forms.

This book is not intended to cover each and every situation that emergency managers might face—remember, each community/jurisdiction is unique and therefore will have different issues to deal with and resolve. The included information, checklists, sample forms, and recommendations in this book are for general guidance only and relate only to those conditions specifically discussed. They should not be considered legal advice for a particular set of circumstances.

# Acknowledgments

I WANT TO EXPRESS MY THANKS to the many emergency management officials and workers that I have met, conversed with, and worked with over the years. My hat is off to all of you for all of your dedication and support. Thanks to my friends Chrystal and John LaPine for all their hard work and encouragement. (These two individuals are the epitome of volunteerism.) There are so many others who have inspired me, such as Tim Murphy, former threat assessment director for the Port of Albany, New York; Jimmy Tuffey, former EM director for the State of New York and current chief of police in Albany, New York; and my many colleagues (Dick, Joe, John, Jodi, Paul, Tom, Eric, Bridget, Kevin, etc.) that I have worked with during many emergency situations in command posts across the country. I appreciate all of you and thank each of you for the experiences we have shared and the lessons that we learned. Thanks to all who have encouraged me on this project and helped in many ways (Sue, Kerrie, Kristen, Jill). A very special thank you goes to my wife, Heather. She has supported me on every undertaking and has also become greatly involved in emergency management herself. This lady is without a doubt my biggest supporter and one who has helped with this project from start to finish. Thank you, honey, for all your support, understanding, and especially your love.

As I often say when dealing with some of the emergency situations we have been involved with over the years, "You can't make this stuff up." Many of you will remember the gold teeth, sneakers, and many other "funnies" that have come up over time. Although it may seem to some that we have way too much fun dealing with disasters, that is simply the way that some of us deal with the stressful atmosphere that often accompanies these events.

# 1

# A History of Emergency Management[1]

A NCIENT PEOPLE RESPONDED TO natural disasters by inventing frameworks to explain the origin of those disasters. This was, in a way, a response, because they saw it as a first step toward preventing future disasters. According to the folklore of the Hawaiian Islands, for example, when the goddess who controlled the volcanoes became angry, she caused molten lava to pour forth from an otherwise quiet mountaintop. Surveys of other cultures reveal parallels; we of course know these frameworks today as myths. Although such supernatural explanations of disasters still exist throughout the world, scientific views of such events have gained ground and are the basis for the modern profession of emergency management.

One of the earliest instances of such efforts was in response to the great fire of London, which struck in 1666. During a 5-day period, 13,200 houses, more than 90 churches, the Royal Exchange, the Customs House, government buildings, and numerous hospitals and libraries burned to the ground. Nearly two-thirds of what was then the world's largest city was destroyed. The losses of 1666 stimulated the gradual adoption of two of the most important forms of nonstructural mitigation ever devised—building codes and insurance. In 1752, nearly a century after the great fire of London, Benjamin Franklin founded the first successful fire insurance company in America.

In 1803, American responses to disasters took a significant turn, starting the pattern of federal involvement that continues today. Following the first of three

---

1. Special thanks to the Tennessee Emergency Management Agency (www.tnema.org) for the use of material for this chapter.

great fires to sweep through Portsmouth, New Hampshire, recovery efforts severely taxed community and state resources. An appeal to Congress brought the first piece of national disaster legislation. Congress responded similarly many times during the following decades.

The greatest disaster in the history of the United States happened in September of 1900, when a hurricane literally submerged Galveston Island, off the coast of Texas. In the city of Galveston alone, at least 6,000 people died, nearly half the homes were swept out of existence, and not a single building went undamaged. Including the destruction outside of the city itself, as many as 12,000 people may have died and well over 3,500 structures destroyed. The Galveston hurricane was a far greater disaster than better-known events such as the Chicago fire of 1871, which killed 250 people; the 1906 San Francisco earthquake, which killed 480; or the Johnstown, Pennsylvania, flood in 1889, which claimed more than 2,200 lives. Between 1803 and 1950, more than one hundred disasters of various types across the nation were fought with federal resources, according to the Federal Emergency Management Agency.

The early years of the twentieth century brought weapons of great destructive power, and the horrors of chemical warfare and civilian bombing in Europe spurred U.S. efforts to organize for civil defense. In 1916, Congress

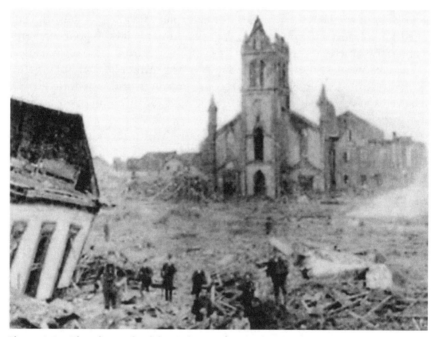

**Figure 1.1.   The aftermath of the Galveston, Texas, hurricane of 1900.**
Courtesy of Freshwater and Marine Image Bank, University of Washington Libraries

enacted the U.S. Army Appropriations Act, the first legislation pertaining to civil defense. This act established the Council of National Defense (CND). The CND established the War Industries Board and encouraged states to create state defense councils. The state councils were encouraged, in turn, to create local defense councils.

In 1939, President Franklin Roosevelt issued a statement on espionage requesting that all citizens, including state and local officials, turn over relevant information to the FBI. The FBI began surveying plants that were under contract to manufacture defense materials and prepared a plant protection manual for use by local police chiefs. (So, even back in the 1930s, state, local and federal law enforcement agencies were working together on various issues.) Shortly after making his espionage statement, Roosevelt established an Office of Emergency Management (OEM). As the world crisis intensified, the coordination responsibilities of the OEM needed to be expanded. For example, the OEM coordinated a wide range of defense-related housing. In 1941, Roosevelt abolished the CND and established the Office of Civil Defense within the Office of Emergency Planning. Like its predecessor, the OCD was linked with what was by then a country-wide system of forty-four state councils and about one thousand local defense councils. Between 1945 and 1949, various government entities examined at civil defense and made recommendations to the president. In 1948, President Harry S. Truman appointed the president of Northwestern Bell Telephone Company to direct the newly formed Office of Civil Defense Planning.

By the early 1950s, there was major shift in civil defense policy. Lots of issues were driving the shift and a government issued report proposed that "... the operational responsibility of civil defense would rest with state and local governments and the federal government would assist in ways it believed to be appropriate." (*Does this sound familiar?*) The report also recommended the establishment of a federal civil defense administration that would report directly to the president of the United States. In December of 1949, President Truman launched the Federal Civil Defense Administration.

Although largely viewed as a creature of the 1950s, "civil defense" had been around for decades. In the course of research for this book, I found many documented references to the protection of the United States against attackers, and even some mentions of state and federal level response to natural disasters as far back as the 1920s. While the protection of the nation itself (that is, the nation's borders) was considered the domain of the federal government, specifically the War Department, response to natural disasters during this period was almost universally the responsibility of local governments.

With respect to the protection of the nation against attackers, there was no organized mechanism for the protection of the civilian population during wars for a great many years, including those fought on American soil (for example, the Civil War). Even after World War I, there was never any concentrated,

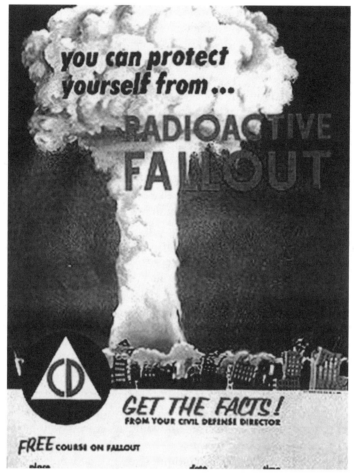

**Figure 1.2.   A Federal Civil Defense Administration poster used in that era.**
Given this backdrop, let's examine some of the specific events that shaped civil defense,
emergency preparedness, and emergency management philosophies and programs at the
local, state, and federal levels within the past fifty years of civil defense and emergency
management in America.

organized attempt to address the protection of the population because it was
largely assumed that no one could launch any significant, direct attacks on the
vast U.S. land mass. The Dust Bowl of the late 1920s and early 1930s saw the first
organized attempts by the federal government to provide some type of "disaster
assistance" to people whose farms had been largely wiped out by the events that
took place during that period.

With the advent of World War II and the fact that, again, all of the battles
and invasions were taking place on the soil of other countries, there still were no

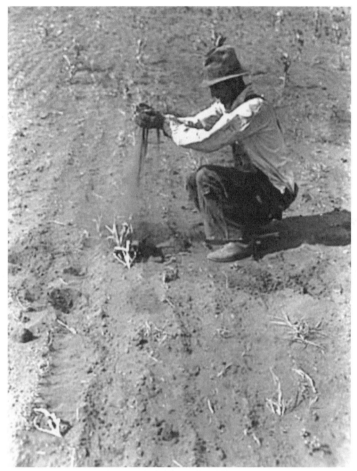

**Figure 1.3.   A farmer during the Dust Bowl years shows that this soil is worthless for growing any crops.**

serious discussions given to civil defense. Following the attack on Pearl Harbor, however, a great many individual communities, especially along the west coast, began to give some serious thought to the possibility of being attacked by aircraft or amphibious forces of Japan. Many of these communities organized civil defense units and issued regulations to outlaw leaving lights on after dark and to allow the reporting of suspicious activities.

Although it happened late in the war, the discovery that Adolf Hitler was developing a missile capable of being launched from a site several hundred miles away would become the first in a series of events that would culminate in the creation of an organized, federal civil defense program. When you combine this with the advent of the atomic bomb development by the United States, the

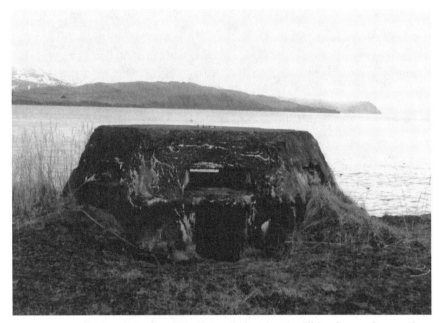

**Figure 1.4.  A bunker from Dutch Harbor, Alaska, that is still in place today. Bunkers such as these were used as lookout points.**

development of long-range bombers, and the subsequent developments in inter-continental missile capabilities, it was not terribly hard to see that there would eventually be a threat to the U.S. homeland. So long as only the United States had these weapons, everything was fairly calm. Once the USSR exploded its first atomic bomb in 1949, however, all bets were off, and there was major concern about the possibility that Russia would eventually attack the United States. Thus, in late 1949, President Harry Truman created the Federal Civil Defense Admin-istration (FCDA).

## The 1950s

On December 1, 1950, President Harry Truman created the Federal Civil De-fense Administration (FCDA) [EO 10186] within what was called the Office of Emergency Management (OEM), attached to the Executive Office of the Presi-dent (EOP). OEM's purpose up to that point had been basically to provide the president with a method to monitor emergencies and disasters that affected the United States, and offered no direct assistance to state or local governments. Congress quickly picked up on this and passed the Federal Civil Defense Act of 1950 [64 Stat. 1245]. On January 12, 1951, the Federal Civil Defense Agency was made an independent agency of the federal government, and absorbed the functions of what had been called the National Security Resources Board (NSRB). The NSRB had been created by the National Security Act of 1947, and was created to "advise the president on mobilization coordination of the United States" during times of war, specifically the buildup of industrial capabilities and the stockpiling of "critical" national security materiel. NSRB also laid the groundwork for the development of CONELRAD, the emergency warning system predecessor to the Emergency Broadcast System (better known to us now as the Emergency Alert System).

Congress passed the Federal Disaster Relief Act, on September 30, 1950, which was designed for the most part to allow the federal government to provide some limited assistance to the states during disaster situations. This function was assigned to the EOP, where it remained (in various forms) until 1973. The Federal Office of Defense Mobilization (ODM) was created by Executive Order (EO) 10193, on December 16, 1950, to coordinate federal mobilization activities (initially for wartime activities), and ODM also inherited the disaster relief coordination responsibilities in another EO (10427), dated January 6, 1953.

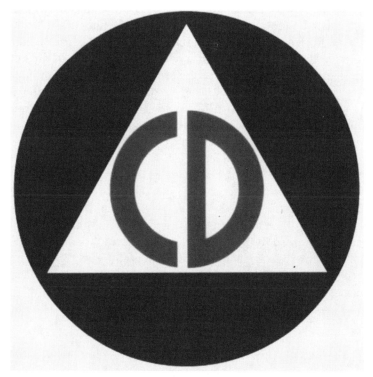

**Figure 1.5. The Civil Defense logo was worn on patches and armbands by Civil Defense workers, who had national security status.**

Do all of these EOs and different agency names and responsibilities have you confused? I'm almost sure that it is confusing to everyone. Just about everyone— at every level of government—was confused during this period also.

The difference between wartime civil defense activities and natural disaster relief activities and their beliefs created friction in many different ways even through the 1980s. Civil Defense (CD) workers were concerned with the protection of the civilian population from the effects of an enemy attack against the country and had "national security" status. Any disaster relief tasks were seen by CD workers as an unrelated, minor task and more or less "not my job."

Initially, Civil Defense programs sought to develop sheltering capabilities to house people living in attacked cities. Civil Defense planners were also developing major evacuation plans for theoretical targets of Russia. Planners naturally assumed that key cities, defense production facilities, and major power plants, among others, would be targeted (*again, does this sound familiar?*) by the Russians in their attempt to take over the continental United States, and began to develop detailed plans for the evacuations of populations from these areas. Comprehensive population and traffic routing studies were undertaken at all levels in an effort to determine how long it would take to evacuate a "targeted" city. Many cities in the country were going to be relocated as part of the overall plan.

In 1953, under yet another reorganization plan, functions of the former NSRB were removed from FCDA and they, along with programs of the existing ODM, FPA, and other disaster and emergency relief responsibilities of the EOP, were consolidated into a new Office of Defense Mobilization, housed within the EOP. The FCDA would concentrate solely on preparing the civilian population for a nuclear attack, while the new ODM would assume all responsibilities related to domestic emergency preparedness and development of the nation's civilian capability to ramp up and go to war. The CONELRAD (alert) program was also transferred to a newly created office called the Assistant Director of Telecommunications, who was to be a part of the new ODM.

In 1958, the major civil defense and emergency preparedness programs at the federal level were reorganized. The FCDA and the ODM were consolidated into a single agency, the Office of Defense and Civilian Mobilization (ODCM), which was to be housed in the Executive Office of the President. It was during this period that the Federal Civil Defense Act was amended to allow the federal government to provide funding for civil emergency preparedness. The federal government provided 50/50 matching funds to personnel and administration costs for agencies engaged in civil defense preparedness.

## 1960s

Despite all of these developments, the general public at large had begun to grow weary of the "duck-and-cover" movie clips and the occasional discussions about civil defense at local community group meetings. People were also realizing that an evacuation of major cities in the event of a nuclear attack was not feasible, so the primary emphasis continued to be centered on fallout shelters.

In 1961, President John F. Kennedy, sensing that the majority of state and local governments were doing little if anything to develop a sheltering capability, decided to make civil defense preparedness a central issue once again. Kennedy separated out "civil defense" functions and other emergency preparedness functions into two agencies. First, he moved the CD functions into and Office of Civil Defense (OCD) within the Department of Defense and assigned responsibility to the Secretary of Defense. A nationwide shelter program, fully funded by the federal government, was developed; it included engineering studies of existing buildings and the acquisition and deployment of shelter stockpiles (the crackers and other nonperishable goods one could find in the basements of these so-designated facilities). This moved "civilian" defense into the military arena, but it was widely believed that the Defense Department had the resources to undertake such a massive logistics program associated with the development of the sheltering program.

Second, what remained of the emergency preparedness programs was transferred to a newly created Office of Emergency Planning (OEP), which became responsible for all civilian emergency preparedness activities, including resource

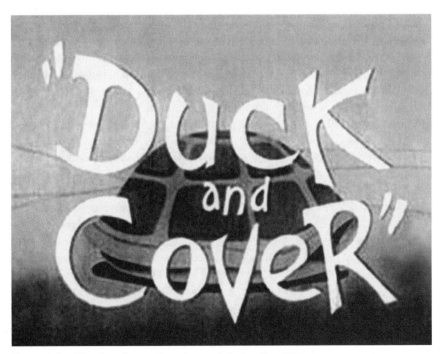

Figure 1.6. "Duck-and-cover" poster used during the 1950s.

utilization, disaster relief, economic stabilization, post-attack rehabilitation, and continuity of government functions. Today, we still have the separation of CD and other emergency functions at the federal level. In 1968, this office was renamed the Office of Emergency Preparedness.

The Cuban Missile Crisis in late 1962 woke everyone up to the renewed possibility of a nuclear attack upon the United States. This incident served to bolster the Defense Department's budget requests for accelerated shelter program development, and this was reflected somewhat in the next budget. Once again, however, the following years would see a dearth of funding for such programs, especially given that—with the removal of missiles from Cuba and the newly developing war in Vietnam—there was once again little interest in the prospect of nuclear attack.

## 1970s

In the early 1970s, under intense pressure from state governors and others who believed that the concept of separated civil defense and emergency preparedness functions was outdated, the federal level organizations moved toward allowing the dual-use of civil defense funds and equipment to be utilized for natural disaster preparedness. In 1971, the OCD was renamed to the Defense Civil Preparedness Agency (DCPA), but retained its basic functions, and the OEP remained intact within the Executive Office of the President. DCPA continued to provide 50/50 matching funds for the "dual-use" concept of civil defense/emergency preparedness at the state and local level. The only visible change at DCPA was that its personnel would now assist state and local governments in developing plans for natural disasters as well as nuclear attacks. Despite the relatively peaceful relationship between the Soviet Union and the United States, the decision was made to maintain a modest civilian defense program.

Reorganization Plan # 1, April 20, 1970, transferred the responsibility for the CONELRAD system to the Office of Telecommunications Policy (OTP) within the EOP. CONELRAD was also renamed the Emergency Broadcast System (EBS). OTP was later absorbed into the Office of Science and Technology Policy, also within the EOP (1978).

On July 1, 1973, Reorganization Plan # 2 took another step backward with the re-delegation of a wide variety of disaster and emergency preparedness activities among a tremendous number of disparate federal agencies. All coordination of federal agency response to major disasters was to be housed at the General Services Administration (GSA), specifically in the Federal Preparedness Agency (FPA), and GSA would also create several other internal divisions for other functions related to emergency preparedness. All coordination of federal disaster relief activities was transferred to the federal Department of Housing and Urban Development (HUD), where it was housed in the Federal Disaster Assistance

Administration. HUD also housed the Federal Insurance Administration (FIA), which had been created in 1968 to provide flood, riot, and crime insurance (in the wake of the race riots of the late 1960s). The Defense Department maintained the DCPA in its original form, largely unchanged by the reorganization plan.

The Federal Fire Prevention and Control Act of 1974 also created two additional emergency preparedness organizations within the Department of Commerce. The National Fire Prevention and Control Administration (NFPCA) was to assist states and localities in the development of fire prevention and control programs, while the National Academy of Fire Prevention and Control (NAFPC) was to develop model training programs for fire service personnel. NFPCA later became the United States Fire Administration in 1978 (still housed in DOC) and the NAFPC and would become the National Fire Academy in that same year.

The 1970s saw a dramatic rise in the number of emergencies and disasters that affected the country's states and localities. The increasing presence of hazardous materials (hazmat) in local communities and in the transportation corridors led to serious hazmat incidents. Chief among them were the bromine release in Rockwood, Tennessee, in 1977 and the LPG explosion in Waverly, Tennessee, in February of 1978. The years 1973–1975 saw dramatic increases in severe weather damages, especially in 1974, where hundreds of people were killed in a series of violent tornado outbreaks across the Midwest. Major flooding events impacted Tennessee in 1977; there were a couple of major dam failures; and the Three Mile Island Nuclear Plant experienced a major malfunction. For a brief period of time, the federal government allowed the states to treat natural disaster preparedness as their primary role with respect to the use of federal civil defense funds. This changed again, however, following the ascendancy of Gerald Ford to the presidency and, once again, states were required to treat planning for a nuclear attack as their primary function, with natural disasters as secondary.

In 1979, President Jimmy Carter created the Federal Emergency Management Agency (FEMA) and consolidated several dozen, disparate emergency preparedness and civil defense functions into a single entity. Although that sounds efficient, many of these organizations continued to function as their own organization within the new agency, and for many years the "civil defense" and "national security" planners were distinct from those that assisted state and local governments in preparing for and responding to disasters. FEMA and its programs would become the basis for state and local emergency preparedness and civil defense programs for the next twenty years.

## 1980s

With the creation of FEMA in 1979, the federal government consolidated several dozen emergency-related programs spread across a multitude of departments into a single entity. Its function was supposed to be the coordination of federal response to disasters and the provision of planning and programmatic assistance to state and local governments in the development of mechanisms to protect the civilian population from all threats. The consolidation of these programs, however, was only cosmetic in nature. Those personnel who had been associated with national security issues remained compartmented, and FEMA directors up through the first Bush administration steered the agency toward "black" and "secret" national security programs, such as continuity of government, relocation of executive branch personnel, and so on. Response to civilian disasters and assistance to state and local governments took a back seat to these programs.

Those within FEMA's civilian programs, however, began to formulate a concept known as "Comprehensive Emergency Management" or CEM. CEM refers to the responsibility for managing response to all types of disasters and emergencies through the coordination of multiple agencies or entities. One of the concepts of CEM was the division of emergency activity into four "phases," specifically mitigation, preparedness, response, and recovery. These phases can be consistently applied across any type of disaster, whether it is manmade, natural, or even attack-related. The Integrated Emergency Management System (IEMS) was also developed during this period. IEMS emphasized the application of "all-hazard" planning for responding to disasters, and FEMA began to allow state and local agencies to focus primarily on natural and technological disasters that affected their communities, and allowed them to relegate nuclear attack planning to the back burner.

In 1984, a methyl isocyante leak in Bophal, India, killed thousands of people and focused attention in the United States on what kinds of chemicals were being stored in local communities. As a result of the Bophal tragedy and several high-profile chemical events that occurred in the United States, the U.S. Congress passed the Superfund Amendments and Reauthorization Act in 1986 (SARA). SARA required any facility that manufactured, used, stored, or processed certain kinds and quantities of chemicals to report information about them to local and state emergency officials, and this information was to be made available to the general public. This would allow community residents to know what kinds of chemicals were being used or stored near their homes, schools, and businesses. Disasters, of course, continued to occur and began to attract much more intense media interest. Major hurricanes such as Hurricane Hugo and earthquakes including those in Loma Prieta (San Francisco) focused attention on the shortcomings in federal assistance to state and local governments. The overwhelming scope of these events focused attention on the need for a federal "response" role—a concept foreign to the recovery role that FEMA had long played. FEMA began work on a Federal Response Plan for a Catastrophic Earthquake in California. Over time, this would evolve into a full-fledged, national government response plan known simply as the Federal Response Plan or FRP. Unfortunately, the FRP had not been implemented prior to the landfall of Hurricane Andrew in 1992. The federal response to this event, perhaps more than any other, focused attention on the need for FEMA to "reinvent" itself.


## 1990s

The 1990s brought with it the "reinvention of government." Perhaps no other agency was more suited to the "poster child" of this concept than FEMA. Upon his appointment as director, James Lee Witt set out to remodel the agency and to make it more attuned to the needs of the state and local governments. FEMA went from being the agency everyone liked to complain about to being one of the more responsive and capable agencies in the federal government—a complete, 180-degree turnaround from the 1992 Hurricane Andrew debacle.

Witt also changed the focus of emergency management so that hazard mitigation was now the foundation of emergency preparedness at all levels of government. Recognizing that it was pointless and costly to simply rebuild homes in areas that flooded every other year, his approach was to provide federal and state funds to buy out homeowners in these areas and turn them into parks, golf courses, and other facilities that, if flooded, suffered little, if any, consequential loss. The theory said that it was much cheaper in the long run to buy out and relocate a homeowner than to have to rebuild his home every other year. This mitigation cornerstone remains in place today.

Director Witt also streamlined the disaster assistance processes of FEMA so that now, when FEMA is called upon to provide temporary housing funds to disaster victims for example, it takes just *a couple of days* to get money to them. This stands in stark contrast to the four to six *weeks* it took just a decade ago. FEMA has also shifted from requiring states to perform certain, specific things in exchange for the funding they receive from the agency, to a program that allows the state to decide which disasters and emergencies affect it most heavily and to develop a program that addresses those issues. This allows the state to concentrate on those types of situations it is most likely to encounter rather than those that are never likely to occur.

Perhaps fittingly, the decade of the 1990s closed out with the most prepared-for nonevent in history—the Y2K "glitch." There was a concern that many of the computer systems in the world that run everything from coffee makers to ATMs to the national defense mechanisms might not be able to interpret the last two zeros in a two-digit date as the year 2000, instead believing it to be 1900. Thousands of "experts" flooded the media preaching gloom and doom and the end of civilization as we knew it. Some people even bought houses way out in the backwoods, stocking them with huge quantities of rations just to be on the safe side in case anarchy ensued. Fortunately, through the dedicated work of thousands of computer professionals, little happened that required the attention of emergency services professionals. The State Emergency Operations Center was activated, however, staffed by about two dozen personnel just in case something did happen. Nothing did, of course, but the staff did enjoy watching the Y2K celebrations from around the globe.

The agency continues to focus on natural and common technological disasters. Today, however, the agency is also forced to focus on such things as domestic preparedness (counterterrorism), critical infrastructure protection (protection of the state's transportation, utility, communications, financial, public health, and governmental systems) and a wide array of other threats that just ten years ago weren't even on the radar scope.

## Timeline

To truly gain an understanding of the highs and lows of civil defense and its evolution into what is now known as emergency management, it is helpful to look back and see how the various agencies that have been assigned related functions have shifted from one department to another, and been renamed, and so on. The Tennessee Emergency Management Agency (TEMA) put together a timeline of the various agencies that managed some aspect of civil defense or emergency management at the federal level. This timeline explores the various organizational entities that preceded the creation of the Federal Emergency Management Agency in 1979. Since FEMA's creation, most of the nation's emergency preparedness functions have remained intact within this one entity for the entire period. Note that many of these changes were simply in name only; many implementations made only cosmetic changes to the function of organization of these groups.

*Coordination of emergency military, civilian, and industrial mobilization; general preparedness planning*

1947–1949   National Security Resources Board, independent entity
1949–1953   NSRB, within the Executive Office of the President (EOP)
1950–1958   Office of Defense Mobilization, EOP
1951–1958   Defense Production Administration, War Department
1958          Office of Defense and Civilian Mobilization, EOP
1958–1961   Office of Civil and Defense Mobilization, EOP
1961–1968   Office of Emergency Planning, EOP
1968–1973   Office of Emergency Preparedness, EOP
1973–1975   Office of Preparedness, General Services Administration
1975–1979   Federal Preparedness Agency, General Services Administration

*Development, operation, and maintenance of emergency telecommunications systems (first CONELRAD, then EBS)*

| | |
|---|---|
| 1951–1953 | National Security Resources Board, independent entity |
| 1951–1953 | Telecommunications Advisor to the President, EOP |
| 1953–1958 | Asst. Director for Telecommunications, Office of Defense Mobilization, EOP |
| 1958 | Asst. Director for Telecommunications, Office of Defense & Civilian Mobilization, EOP |
| 1958–1961 | Asst. Director for Telecommunications, Office of Civil & Defense Mobilization, EOP |
| 1961–1968 | Asst. Director for Telecommunications, Office of Emergency Planning, EOP |
| 1968–1970 | Asst. Director for Telecommunications, Office of Emergency Preparedness, EOP |
| 1970–1978 | Office of Telecommunications Policy, EOP |
| 1978–1979 | Office of Science and Technology Policy, EOP (EBS oversight only) |

*Administration of Civil Defense programs*

| | |
|---|---|
| 1950–1951 | Federal Civil Defense Administration, EOP |
| 1951–1958 | Federal Civil Defense Administration, independent entity |
| 1958 | Office of Defense and Civilian Mobilization, EOP |
| 1958–1961 | Office of Civil and Defense Mobilization, EOP |
| 1961–1972 | Office of Civil Defense, Department of the Army |
| 1972–1979 | Defense Civil Preparedness Agency |

*Administration of disaster assistance and insurance programs*

| | |
|---|---|
| 1953–1958 | Office of Defense Mobilization, EOP |
| 1958 | Office of Defense and Civilian Mobilization, EOP |
| 1958–1961 | Office of Civil and Defense Mobilization, EOP |
| 1961–1968 | Office of Emergency Planning, EOP |
| 1968–1973 | Office of Emergency Preparedness, EOP |
| 1973–1979 | Federal Disaster Assistance Administration, Dept. of Housing and Urban Development |
| 1968–1979 | Federal Insurance Administration, Dept. of Housing and Urban Development |

*Administration of fire prevention and training programs*

| | |
|---|---|
| 1974–1978 | National Fire Prevention and Control Administration, Dept. of Commerce |

1974–1978   National Academy of Fire Prevention and Control
                    Dept. of Commerce
1978–1979   U. S. Fire Administration, Department of Commerce

*Consolidation of federal disaster assistance, emergency planning, fire and emergency management training, and insurance programs*

1979   EO 12127, March 31, 1979, created the Federal Emergency
           Management Agency

One of the things many people remember about the "civil defense" era was the public fallout shelter signs that were posted on many buildings in just about every city in the country. While these and the CD seal image were everywhere during the 1950s through 1970s, there are many posters, training manuals, advertisements, and other documents bearing the images that, while some people have seen them, many have not.

# 2

# Emergency Management
# and the All-Hazards Approach

"Disaster: a calamitous event causing great loss of life, damage, or hardship."

—*Black's Law Dictionary*

EMERGENCY MANAGEMENT and preparedness incorporate the areas of emergency, risk, disaster, and hazard management in addition to aspects of civil defense and protection. While some of these terms are synonymous to some extent (especially *emergency* and *disaster*), let me give you some of my personal definitions. My definition of *emergency* is "an extraordinary event that goes beyond the capacity of normal resources and the typical organization to cope with." All emergencies are by definition dangerous, which means that injury and/or the potential loss of life is involved. We can break down emergencies to four levels:

- Routine problem—the most minor of emergencies, usually involving first responders
- Incident—any emergency a community can handle without calling in outside help
- Disaster—an incident involving extensive damage and likely mass casualties
- National (or international) disaster—a disaster of significant scale and seriousness

Emergency management can be done by more than one individual, but it is probably most ideally done by one individual. Good emergency management seeks to reduce improvisation to the absolute minimum, and good emergency

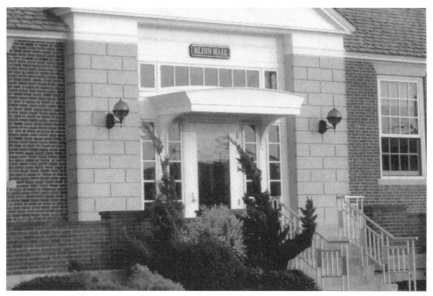

**Figure 2.1.   Massachusetts Maritime Academy has a graduate degree program in emergency management.**

managers tend to be persons with years of education, experience, and training. Current hazard and disaster management, usually associated with the emergency preparedness field, as that field has evolved from the old civil defense days to an all-hazards approach, also has certain personnel demands. There is a progressive upgrading of qualifications to become a manager, planner, or director in all emergency-related fields. Many colleges and universities are now offering a graduate-level program in emergency management; Massachusetts Maritime Academy is one such school (see its website at www.maritime.edu).

### Emergency Management Directors

Most state directors of emergency management hold appointed, political positions. In twenty-seven out of fifty states, they are appointed directly by the governor, and in seventeen other states, appointment is by a state cabinet-level official. In the remaining six states, the director of emergency management is a merit-based, civil-service position. Since 9/11, about ten states have made their emergency management director the single point of contact for homeland security in that state; while the other forty states have seen fit to create whole new state-level commissioners, directors, superintendents, or secretaries of homeland security. According to the National Emergency Managers Association (www .nemaweb.org), the average state emergency management director is a fifty-five-year-old man who holds at least a bachelor's degree and makes approximately $75,000 per year, is appointed by the governor and reports to the adjutant general, has been in the position an average of four years, and supervises an average of three presidential and five gubernatorial disaster declarations per year. On average, the disaster budget for each state is about $53 million (some large states have upwards of $637 million) and the number of employees averages 62 (with some states having upwards of 512 employees).

## The All-Hazards Approach and the Four Phases of Comprehensive Emergency Management

While emergency managers can't foretell what emergency situations will occur, they can certainly prepare for them. There are many kinds of emergency events that can affect a community, including fires, natural disasters, and manmade crises. Ideally, an emergency manager would have a detailed, operating procedure in place for every possibility—but, in reality, it is nearly impossible to have a plan for every type of emergency that may occur.

Assessing the possible threats to a city, town, or state quickly adds up to a lengthy list of potential hazards. Emergency managers can identify areas of vulnerability by considering factors both internal and external to the locale. Communities that have facilities that store and use hazardous materials, for example, should be prepared to deal with a potential spill, leak, or release. Communities that exist in the path of frequent hurricanes can benefit from the reinforcement that specialized building materials provide.

Yet, planning for known vulnerabilities is only part of the picture that emergency managers must deal with. As we see on the news reports and read about almost on a daily basis, a community can be affected by an assortment of threats, from a fire to a tornado to a terrorist attack. The plan that takes into account the various threats and circumstances that communities can face is one designed with what we call an all-hazards approach.

The Federal Emergency Management Agency (FEMA) suggests that emergency management agencies use an all-hazards approach in their emergency preparedness policies. An *all-hazards approach* is based on the idea that the community's emergency plan follows the same philosophies and actions no matter what the emergency situation. What this means is that the plan sets up a distinct, all-inclusive structure for the management of emergency incidents and uses consistent procedures and policies.

There are four phases of Comprehensive Emergency Management (CEM), and these formulate the basis for the all-hazards approach to emergency management. The four phases are mitigation, preparedness, response, and recovery.

- Mitigation includes efforts to prevent manmade or natural disasters by the assessment of threats to a community. These assessments include the likelihood of an attack or disaster taking place.
- Preparedness includes the planning, resource allocation, and training of individuals. This phase also has disaster response exercises that help people practice what to do if a disaster occurs.
- Response includes public donations, incident management, coordination, search and rescue operations, damage assessments, and handling of fatalities.
- Recovery involves cleaning up, the reinstitution of public services, the rebuilding of public infrastructure, and all that is necessary to help restore civic life, including disaster assistance and crisis counseling.

### Risk Analysis

The first step in any emergency or disaster planning is to identify the risks. Risks are not the same as perils, which are a cause of risk; neither should risk be confused with hazards, which are contributing factors to peril. Almost anything can be a *hazard* (an extension cord on the ground, for example) and any sort of life-threatening disaster can be a *peril* (such as a fire, earthquake, or hurricane), but *risk* technically refers to something that can be measured and always involves a loss or at least a decrease in the value of some assets. Examples of risk include pesticide poisoning, hazardous waste, auto accidents, death by firearms, weapons of mass destruction, and radiation exposure. Note how in each case, the risk usually involves something you have to do (eradicate pests) which is the benefit, and something you wish didn't have to accompany the benefit (the cost, or potential poisoning of crops).

Two other terms also need defining: *threat,* which is anything adversely affecting an asset (and threats can be natural, accidental, or intentional); and *vulnerability,* which is any weakness or flaw than can conceivably be exploited by a threat. Threat assessment is usually the first step in the overall risk-assessment process; threat assessment is normally concerned with the credibility and/or nonrandomness of the threat. The next step is usually vulnerability assessment, which normally ranks the expected losses from impact. The next step of risk analysis usually integrates these impact or loss ratings with vulnerability ratings to produce a matrix for the cost-benefit evaluation of various countermeasures.

Since risks vary from community to community, it is important to adapt planning and preparedness for each location. There is no "silver bullet" emergency plan for all locations, unfortunately. In the process of identifying all the risks, emergency managers need to look at worst-case scenario assessments based on various what-if questions. There are no set guidelines for how in depth these assessments should be—but, generally, we need to keep in mind the realistic chances of prevention and other protective efforts. Certain standard hazards exist that can serve as starting points in any risk analysis. We look now at two types of hazards: natural and technological.

- Natural disasters are naturally occurring; examples are earthquakes, volcanic eruptions, hurricanes, tornados, ice storms, floods, flashfloods, landslides, wildfires, insect infestation, and disease outbreaks.
- Technological disasters are those associated with scientific, industrial, or electronic advances; examples are explosives, unexploded ordnance, toxic spills, emissions of radio-isotopes, terrorism, and transportation accidents. Other examples include hazmat incidents involving carcinogens, mutagens, or heavy metals; and dangerous processes, especially involving the structural failure of devices, machines, installations, or plants—such as bridges, dams, mines, power plants, pipelines, high rise buildings, vehicles, and trains.

Table 2.1 includes the basic elements of an emergency plan. This plan can be modified to fit your community's needs.

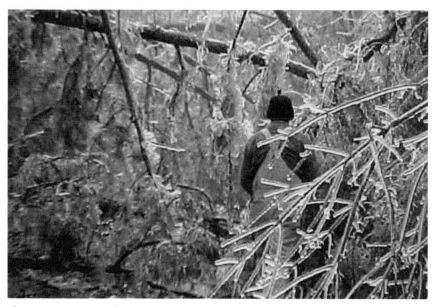

**Figure 2.2.    A severe ice storm can cause a great deal of damage.**

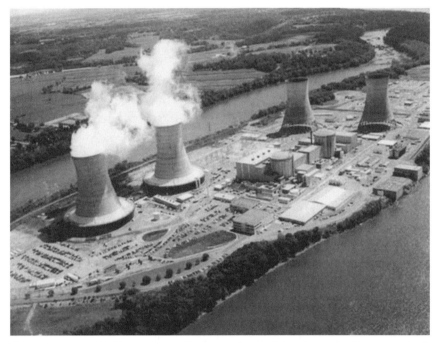

**Figure 2.3   Powers plants are sometimes associated with technological advances leading to technological disasters.**

**TABLE 2.1**
**Elements of an Emergency Plan**

1. Title
2. Preface: jurisdictions, sponsorship, authorities involved, dates
3. Introduction
    3.1. Policy statement by Chief Executive Officer (mayor, administrator, etc.)
    3.2. Legislative authority for the design of the plan
    3.3. General purpose of the plan
    3.4. Conditions under which the plan will be used
    3.5. National and regional framework of local emergency planning
4. Local hazards
    4.1. Types of local risks
    4.2. Description of local area, its characteristics, resources, and hazards
    4.3. Historical description of impacts (any previous disasters, etc.)
5. Vulnerability and risk analysis of local population, built environment, economic activities, social and cultural systems
    5.1. Assessment of community disaster probabilities
    5.2. Risk analysis (hazard × vulnerability × exposure)
    5.3. Risk and disaster scenarios for the local area
    5.4. Risk-management strategies
6. Legal and jurisdictional responsibilities for emergency management
    6.1. Including warning, evacuation, search and rescue, and healthcare and sanitation
7. Introduction to local emergency management resources
    7.1. Personnel, equipment, supplies, communications, shelters, etc.

8. Structure of local emergency command system
   8.1. Authority organization chart
   8.2. Organizational relationships, coordination and command structures, mutual-aid agreements, and relations with other jurisdictions
   8.3. Relationships with other levels of government, particularly emergency-related agencies
9. General all-hazards plan or plans for specific types of emergency
   9.1. Roles, relationships, and tasks
      9.1.1. Operation of warning systems
         9.1.1.1. Types of warnings, how they will be distributed, obligations on receiving warnings
      9.1.2. Pre-impact preparations
         9.1.2.1. Relationships between type of disaster agent and necessary preparations
         9.1.2.2. Responsibilities of different agencies
         9.1.2.3. Location of sites of greatest risk
      9.1.3. Emergency evacuation procedures
         9.1.3.1. Conditions under which evacuation is authorized
         9.1.3.2. Routes to be followed and destinations
         9.1.3.3. How the special needs of the elderly, ill, physically challenged, or institutionalized will be accommodated
         9.1.3.4. Locations of emergency shelters (maps included)
      9.1.4. Emergency-operations centers and incident-command centers
         9.1.4.1. Locations, equipment, operations, and staffing
      9.1.5. Communications
      9.1.6. Search and rescue (SAR)
         9.1.6.1. Responsibilities, equipment, and places most likely to require SAR work
      9.1.7. Public order
      9.1.8. Public information (media)
         9.1.8.1. Management of the mass media
      9.1.9. Medical facilities and morgues
         9.1.9.1. Location, transportation, capacity, and facilities
      9.1.10. Restoration of basic services: order of priorities, responsibilities
         9.1.10.1. Protection against continuing threat
         9.1.10.2. The search for secondary threats, actions to be taken if discovered
         9.1.10.3. Continuing assessment of the total situation: responsibilities, distribution
10. Plans for specific sections
    10.1. Airports, hospitals, museums, secure institutions, archives, tourism, factories, nuclear reactors, schools, etc.
11. Arrangements for testing, disseminating, and updating the plan
    11.1. Plan distribution and publicity
    11.2. Field exercises and their evaluation
    11.3. Standard or automatic procedures for updating the plan
12. Appendices
    12.1. Tables of data
    12.2. Maps and photographs
    12.3. Lists of names, addresses, and contact numbers of all relevant agencies, their heads, and deputies
    12.4. Detailed descriptions and strategies

## Emergency Operations Center

An Emergency Operations Center (EOC) should be a well-thought-out and well-equipped room or building. Many emergency managers may not fully understand the structure and functions of an EOC in today's era of terrorism where the need for communication (with both the public and political leaders) is so critical. As an example, in the case of a bioterrorism incident, the EOC would have to put together politics and law for matters like:

- Quarantine
- Inoculations (smallpox)
- Forced evacuation
- Any other matters affecting citizens' rights

Also, in disasters of great magnitude, many multiple jurisdictional personnel are operating in the same jurisdiction simultaneously. Hazmat teams and special rescue teams normally have with their own command structure in place. Medical teams typically come with their own legal authority. The problem of "who's in charge" is usually resolved where the highest-ranking elected official in the local jurisdiction is in charge, unless another rule or standard is in place or until that default person passes the command function to someone else who is qualified.

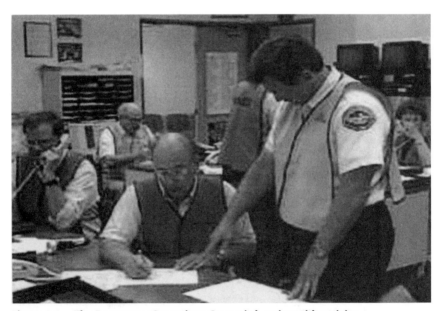

**Figure 2.4.   The Emergency Operations Center is buzzing with activity.**

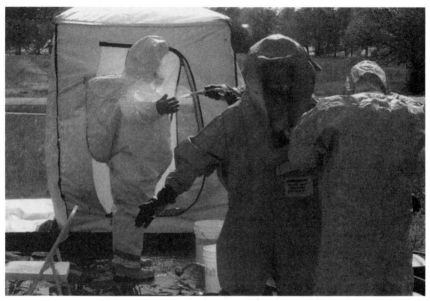

**Figure 2.5  A hazardous material team undergoing decontamination.**

An EOC should have the following characteristics:

- Location: The EOC needs to occupy a location well connected in terms of telecommunications and in terms of accessibility by roads and possibly rail or air terminals. The site should be safe from hazards (for example, it should not be floodable or located on unstable ground) and the building should be resistant to wind damage, water penetration, earthquake shaking, or whatever the plan deals with in terms of hazards. It is wise to place the EOC close to critical emergency facilities, such as a fire station or ambulance center. Although most communication will be by radio or telephone, face-to-face consultation may still be a necessary way of clarifying difficult problems. The EOC should be easily recognized and identified by large signs on its principal facades. However, it should not be easily accessible to casual visitors.
- Communications: The EOC should be sufficiently supplied with telephone, fax, Internet, and radio transmitter equipment and connections. The level of investment in these will obviously depend on the budget, the size of the emergency services to be directed, and the extent and population size of the area to be covered.
- Equipment and facilities: The EOC will require various other facilities, according to the scale of operation. These include computer/printer equipment and software, including computer display equipment for large-scale displays of shared data and maps, a geographic information system (GIS)

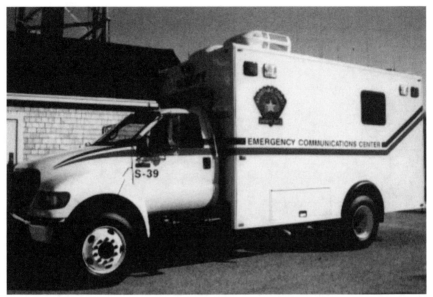

**Figure 2.6.   Oftentimes, a mobile communications unit is called to supplement the EOC's communications abilities.**

for the analysis of local site conditions, and emergency management and communications programs. Television and radio receivers are essential to have in order to view the news media's treatment of evolving disasters; since often the general public will be managed on the basis of what messages have been broadcast, it will be necessary to monitor both these reports and the public's reactions to them. I would suggest the capability of recording the media if at all possible (VCR, DVD, DVR). A well-equipped EOC will have stocks of food and drinks, limited cooking and sleeping facilities, and supplies of tools and protective clothing. These are not for the benefit of victims or emergency workers, but are intended to help guarantee the EOC a level of independence when disaster strikes and work shifts are greatly prolonged. Finally, it is useful to have plenty of parking spaces in the vicinity of the EOC so that emergency vehicles and supplies can be assembled and loaded/unloaded during drills, exercises, and actual disasters.

- Media-briefing facilities: The EOC should have a conference room or JIC (Joint Information Center) where information can be given to journalists and where interviews can be conducted for radio and television. This room will require audiovisual equipment and other appropriate aids, such as a podium and a backdrop with the agency's logo on it. Office space for reporters and communications facilities for the media may also be provided in some of the larger EOCs. Keep media away from the actual workspace of the EOC.
- Instructional facilities: Some EOCs have rooms with blackboards, multimedia projectors, and other projection equipment. This means that they can

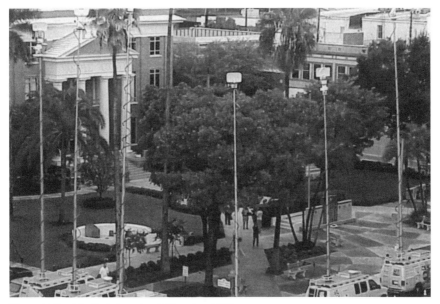

Figure 2.7. Media interest outside of an EOC.

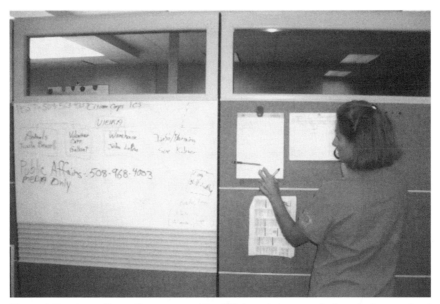

Figure 2.8. A small meeting room, with whiteboard, is a good place to have a short meeting.

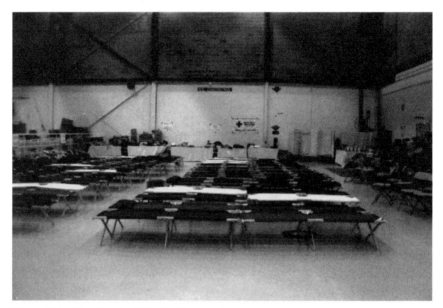

**Figure 2.9.   Sleeping facilities (cots) are set up.**

be used for training sessions, seminars, and planning meetings. At the least, it is helpful to have a small conference room in which heads of emergency services, scientists, and political and community leaders can get together and confer on tactics as conditions change during emergencies.

## Work Cited

*Black's Law Dictionary*, 7th Edition (St. Paul, MN: West Publishing Company, 1999), p. 475.

# 3

# The National Incident Management System (NIMS) and the Incident Command System (ICS)

T HE NATIONAL INCIDENT MANAGEMENT SYSTEM (NIMS) is the first-ever standardized approach to incident management and response. Developed by the Department of Homeland Security (DHS) and released in March of 2004, NIMS establishes a uniform set of methods and procedures that emergency responders at all levels of government will use to conduct response operations. Developed by the Secretary of Homeland Security at the request of the president, the National Incident Management System also combines effective practices in emergency response into a comprehensive national framework for incident management. The NIMS will enable responders at all levels to work together more effectively and efficiently to manage incidents no matter what the cause, size, or complexity, including disasters and catastrophic acts such as terrorism.

Federal agencies are also required to use the NIMS framework in domestic incident management and in support of state and local incident response and recovery activities, when requested to do so.

The benefits of the NIMS system are noteworthy, and include the following:

- Standardized organizational structures, processes, and procedures;
- Standards for planning, training, and exercising;
- Personnel qualification standards;
- Equipment acquisition and certification standards;
- Interoperable communications processes, procedures, and systems;
- Information management systems with a commonly accepted style;
- Supporting technologies—voice and data communications systems, information systems, data display systems, specialized technologies; and
- Publication management processes and activities.

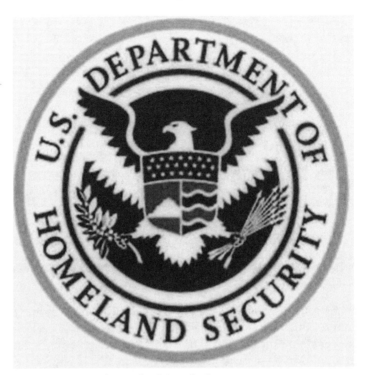

**Figure 3.1.   Department of Homeland Security logo.**

Government agencies within the Department of Homeland Security will be developing additional NIMS compliance guidance in the future; communities and other jurisdictions will be provided with some resources to help them through the NIMS compliance process.

NIMS should be seen as a living document that will require continuous maintenance by the jurisdictions implementing it. When new guidelines or compliance issues arise, it will likely fall to the emergency manager to ensure full compliance.

It is often asked if the adoption of NIMS is a requirement for Department of Homeland Security funding. As mandated by Homeland Security Presidential Directive-5 (HSPD-5), beginning in Fiscal Year (FY) 2005, adoption of NIMS will be a condition for receiving federal preparedness funds, including grants, contracts, and other activities, including training, drills, and exercises. So, the answer to the question is yes, adoption of NIMS is a requirement.

For the time being, communities/jurisdictions will be considered to be in compliance with the NIMS by adopting the Incident Command System (ICS) and NIMS principles and policies. Other aspects of the NIMS will require additional development and refinement to enable compliance at a future date. See appendix E for a sample city/town ordinance.

The NIMS will eventually ensure interoperability of equipment and communications and the certification of emergency response and incident management personnel. This means there will be the development of standardized criteria for the qualification, training, and certification of response personnel. NIMS will also make possible the development of a system of typed and categorized resources, to include equipment, teams and personnel.

As stated earlier, HSPD-5 required federal departments and agencies to make adoption of NIMS by state and local organizations a condition for federal preparedness assistance by FY 2005. Organizations and personnel at all governmental levels and in the private sector must be trained to improve all-hazard incident management capability. These organizations and personnel must also participate in realistic (and periodic) exercises to improve integration and interoperability.

Under NIMS, preparedness is based on national standards for qualification and certification of emergency response personnel. Managed by the NIMS Integration Center (NIC), standards will help ensure that the participating agencies' and organizations' field personnel possess (at least) the minimum knowledge, skills, and experience required to perform their activities safely and effectively. The standards will include training, experience, and credentialing, as well as physical and medical fitness. Personnel who are certified to support interstate incidents will be required to meet national qualification and certification standards.

The Emergency Management Institute (a DHS/FEMA agency specializing in emergency management training) has developed several Web-based courses dealing with many emergency management topics. They also have a course entitled "The National Incident Management System, an Introduction." This course, and all Web-based training from EMI, is available free of charge to U.S. residents via the FEMA training website.

The course describes the purpose, principles, key components, and benefits of NIMS. Also included in the course are online "Planning Activity" tools that help users to measure how compliant their organization is with NIMS.

After completing the IS 700 course, participants will be able to:

- Describe the key concepts and principles underlying NIMS;
- Identify the benefits of using ICS as the national incident management model;
- Describe when it is appropriate to institute an Area Command;
- Describe when it is appropriate to institute a Multi-Agency Coordination System;
- Describe the benefits of using a Joint Information System (JIS) for public information;

- Identify the ways in which NIMS affects preparedness;
- Describe how NIMS affects how resources are managed;
- Describe the advantages of common communication and information management systems;
- Explain how NIMS influences technology and technology systems; and
- Describe the purpose of the NIMS Integration Center.

The NIC has developed a National Mutual Aid Glossary of Terms and Definitions as well as Resource Typing Definitions for some of the most commonly used resources during a response. *Resource typing* is an integral component of the National Incident Management System. It enhances the ability of emergency responders to find needed resources during a disaster. In compliance with NIMS and in support of the Incident Command System (ICS), the Resource Typing Definitions and Mutual Aid Glossary of Terms and Definitions also help promote common terminology of descriptions, standards, and types of local, state, and federal response assets.

Resource typing definitions provide emergency managers with the information they need to request and receive the resources they need during an emergency or disaster. The National Mutual Aid Glossary and the Resource Typing Definitions will be continuously updated, revised, and expanded as needed.

### The National Mutual Aid and Resource Management System

The National Mutual Aid and Resource Management System is an initiative undertaken by the Department of Homeland Security through the NIMS Integrations Center and the Federal Emergency Management Agency, in cooperation with the National Emergency Management Association (NEMA). This system will enhance emergency readiness and response at all levels of government through a comprehensive and integrated system that will allow a jurisdiction to augment response resources, if needed. The system will allow emergency management personnel to identify, locate, request, order, and track outside resources quickly and effectively. It will allow them to obtain information on specific resource capabilities, locations, costs, and support requirements.

The key concepts of the National Mutual Aid and Resource Management System include:

- The use of pre-incident agreements (including mutual aid, Emergency Management Assistance Compact (EMAC), and others) by donor and requesting jurisdictions;
- Protocols for documenting and inventorying disaster response resources in terms of categories, kinds, components, metrics, and typing definitions;

- A national deployable inventory of pre-identified credentialed, categorized, and capability-typed resources. These resources would be entered into the system voluntarily by federal, state, tribal, or local authorities, nongovernment institutions, and/or private sector entities participating in mutual-aid disaster response operations; and
- An Automated Resource Management System (ARMS) to access and search the inventory/catalog to locate, request, order, and track resources requested by incident management personnel in need of assistance.

## The Incident Command System

ICS is a standardized on-scene incident management concept designed specifically to allow responders to adopt an integrated organizational structure equal to the complexity and demands of any single incident or multiple incidents without being hindered by jurisdictional boundaries.

In the early 1970s, ICS was developed to manage rapidly moving wildfires in California and to address the following problems:

- Too many people reporting to one supervisor;
- Different emergency response organizational structures;
- Lack of reliable incident information;
- Inadequate and incompatible communications;
- Lack of structure for coordinated planning among agencies;
- Unclear lines of authority; and
- Terminology differences among and between agencies.

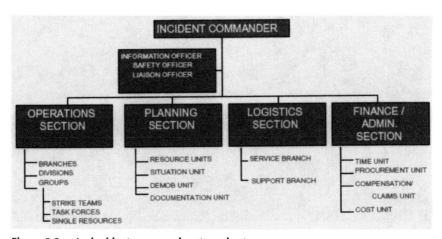

Figure 3.2.   An incident command system chart.

In 1980, federal officials transitioned ICS into a national program called the National Interagency Incident Management System (NIIMS), which became the basis of a response management system for all federal agencies with wildfire management responsibilities. Since then, most federal (and state and local) agencies have endorsed the use of ICS and have mandated its use.

An Incident Command System enables integrated communication and planning by establishing a manageable span of control. Additionally, an ICS divides an emergency response into five manageable functions essential for emergency response operations: Command, Operations, Planning, Logistics, and Finance and Administration.

## Unified Command (UC)

Although a single incident commander normally handles the command function, an Incident Command System organization may be expanded into a Unified Command (UC). The UC is a structure that brings together the incident commanders of all major organizations involved in the incident, in order to coordinate an effective response while at the same time allowing them to carry out their own jurisdictional responsibilities. The UC links the organizations responding to the incident and provides a forum for these entities to make con-

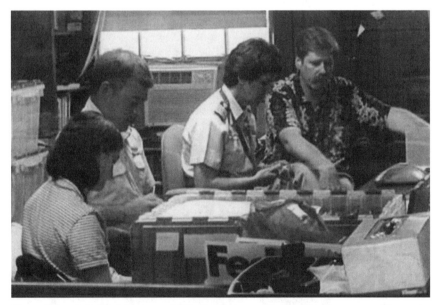

Figure 3.3.   A Unified Command Meeting between the USCG, the responsible party, and the State of Massachusetts.

sensus decisions. Under the UC, the various jurisdictions and/or agencies and nongovernment responders may blend together throughout the operation to create an integrated response team.

The UC is responsible for overall management of the incident. The UC directs incident activities, including development and implementation of overall objectives and strategies, and approves ordering and releasing of resources. Members of the UC work together to develop a common set of incident objectives and strategies, share information, maximize the use of available resources, and enhance the efficiency of the individual response organizations.

## NIMS and ICS

The NIMS utilizes ICS as a standard incident management organization for the management of all major incidents. These functional areas include command, operations, planning, logistics, and finance/administration. Additionally, the principle of unified command has been incorporated into NIMS to ensure further coordination for incidents involving multiple jurisdictions and/or agencies. This unified command component not only coordinates the efforts of many jurisdictions, but also provides for and assures joint decision making on objectives, strategies, plans, priorities, and communications to and with the public.

The NIMS recognizes the National Wildfire Coordinating Group (NWCG) ICS training as a model for course curricula and materials applicable to the NIMS:

- ICS-100, Introduction to ICS
- ICS-200, Basic ICS
- ICS-300, Intermediate ICS
- ICS-400, Advanced ICS

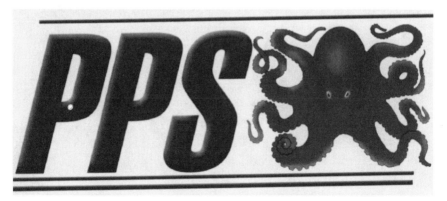

Figure 3.4.   The PPS logo.

The National Fire Academy and the Emergency Management Institute both follow this model in their ICS training curricula. At the local level, agencies may contact their state fire academy or emergency management agency for information and training on ICS. Some private entities, such as Precision Planning and Simulation (PPS) (see www.ppscorp.com), also provide ICS training.

## Mutual-Aid Agreements

Mutual-aid agreements are the means for one jurisdiction to provide resources, facilities, services, personnel, and other required support to another jurisdiction during an incident. Each jurisdiction should be party to a mutual-aid agreement (such as the Emergency Management Assistance Compact) with appropriate jurisdictions from which they expect to receive or to which they expect to provide assistance during an incident. This would normally include all neighboring or nearby jurisdictions, as well as relevant private-sector and nongovernmental organizations. Many states participate in interstate compacts and also have established intrastate agreements that encompass all local jurisdictions. Mutual-aid

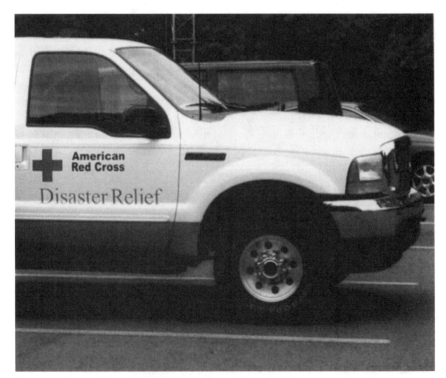

**Figure 3.5. A Red Cross vehicle parked at a disaster site.**

agreements may also be needed with private organizations such as the American Red Cross, Salvation Army, and others to facilitate the timely delivery of private assistance at the appropriate level during incidents.

At a minimum, mutual-aid agreements should include the following elements or provisions:

- Definitions of key terms used in the agreement;
- Roles and responsibilities of individual parties;
- Procedures for requesting and providing assistance;
- Procedures, authorities, and rules for payment, reimbursement, and allocation of costs;
- Notification procedures;
- Protocols for interoperable communications;
- Relationships with other agreements among jurisdictions;
- Workers' compensation;
- Treatment of liability and immunity;
- Recognition of qualifications and certifications; and
- Sharing agreements, as required.

Authorized officials from each of the participating jurisdictions need to jointly approve all mutual-aid agreements.

The concept of regional mutual aid is based on consistency and simplicity and is borne out of the prospect of a large-scale incident (such as a major natural event or large-scale terrorist event) involving multiple jurisdictions in the response. Coordination of resources and response personnel across multiple counties will be more effective if similar agreements are in place, expectations are consistent, and reimbursement procedures have been negotiated with regional input prior to an event.

### Community Involvement

NIMS compliance should be considered and undertaken as a community-wide effort. The benefit of NIMS is most apparent at the local level, when a community as a whole prepares for and provides an integrated response to an incident. Incident response organizations—to include local departments of public health, public works, emergency management, fire, emergency medical services, law enforcement, and hazardous materials, and private sector entities, nongovernmental organizations, medical organizations, utility companies, as well as others—need to work together to comply with the various NIMS components, policies, and procedures. Implementation of the NIMS in every local jurisdiction establishes a baseline capability. Once communities establish that baseline, it can be used

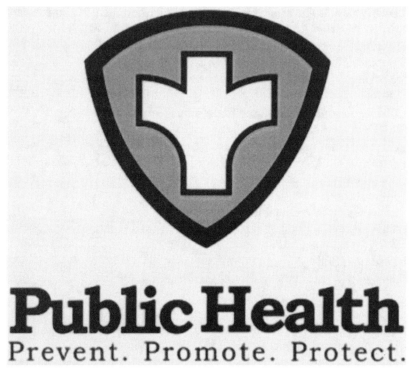

**Figure 3.6 The new Public Health logo.**

as a foundation upon which more advanced emergency planning and homeland security capabilities can be built on a national scale.

In many instances smaller (rural) communities may not have the resources to implement all elements of NIMS on their own. On the other hand, by working together with other localities in their regions, these jurisdictions will be able to pool their resources, saving valuable tax dollars, to implement NIMS. Even though many larger communities do have the resources, and perhaps the money to implement all of the elements of NIMS, it makes good sense to use this same concept of pooling resources with other communities.

## Summary

As an emergency manager, it is important to realize that when NIMS is fully implemented, your local community or jurisdiction will be able to:

- Ensure common and proven incident management practices and principles that are used to plan for, protect against, respond to, and recover from an emergency incident. The concepts of the NIMS are also effective in planning and conducting pre-planned events (parades, festivals, dignitary visits, and so on);

- Maintain a response operation capable of expanding to meet an escalating situation and the ability to integrate resources and equipment from intrastate and interstate mutual-aid agreements, state-provided assistance, and federal government response;
- Request and track response assets using common resource typing and definitions, and draw on mutual-aid agreements for additional assistance, as needed;
- Establish staging and allocation plans for the redistribution of equipment, supplies, and resources coming into the area from other localities, states, or the federal government through mutual-aid agreements;
- Conduct situational assessments and establish the appropriate Incident Command System organizational structure to effectively manage the incident;
- Establish communication processes, procedures, and protocols that will ensure effective interoperable communications among emergency responders, 911 centers, and multi-agency coordination systems (Emergency Operations Centers). This will include the use of common terminology and plain language (no codes).

The NIMS is much more than just a list of elements required of communities and jurisdictions by the federal government. It is a whole new approach to the way we as emergency managers prepare for and manage incidents. It is an approach that will hopefully lead to a more effective use of resources and improved prevention, preparedness, and response capabilities. In addition, full NIMS implementation is a dynamic and multi-year phase-in process with important linkages to the National Response Plan (NRP), the Homeland Security Presidential Directive 8 (the "National Preparedness Goal"), and the National Infrastructure Protection Plan (NIPP). I am quite sure that future fine-tuning of the NIMS will grow as policy and technical issues are further developed and clarified at the national level.

# 4

# Natural Hazards

Natural hazards are defined as those particular hazard events that arise from geophysical processes or biological agents and affect the lives, livelihood, or the property of the public. They include:

- Ice and snowstorms
- Thunderstorms
- Lightning
- Tornadoes
- Hailstorms
- Windstorms
- Extreme temperatures (both hot and cold)
- Flooding
- Drought
- Wildfires
- Infectious diseases
- Earthquakes

Each of these natural hazards presents a unique challenge with respect to the response by the emergency manager.

## Ice and Snowstorms

Ice and snowstorms are those occasions when damaging accumulations of ice or snow take place during freezing rain/snow situations. The terms *freezing rain/*

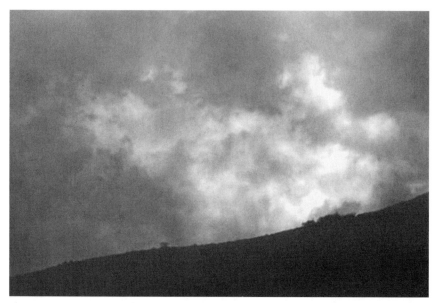

**Figure 4.1.** A large wildfire in California.

**Figure 4.2.** A large tornado.

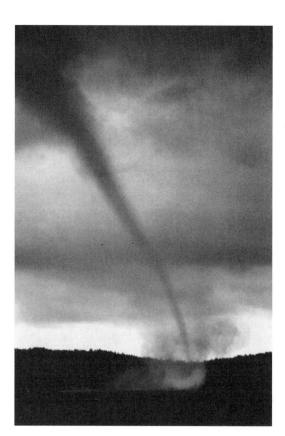

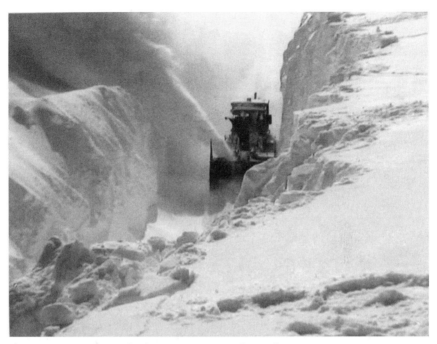

Figure 4.3. Snowstorm in the upstate New York area in 2007.

*snow* and *freezing drizzle* are usually sufficient to warn the general public that a coating of ice and an accumulation of snow is expected on the ground and other exposed streets and surfaces, making travel and other activities difficult. A heavy accumulation of ice or snow can bring down trees, electrical wires, telephone poles and lines, and even communication towers, putting a great strain on public safety and the general public's ability to communicate and travel.

Power and communications can sometimes be disrupted for several days while utility companies work to repair the often-extensive damage. Utility companies often have to bring in assistance from outside the affected area, and that takes time and coordination. Ice forming on exposed surfaces generally ranges from a thin glaze to coatings of approximately one-inch thick or more. Snowfalls and drifts can range from a slight dusting to several feet, depending on the part of the country. The even-smaller accumulations of ice on sidewalks, streets, and highways may cause extreme hazards for community residents, motorists, pedestrians, and the first responder population.

Sleet does not stick to trees and wires. However, sleet in sufficient depth does cause treacherous driving conditions and this often results in many major motor vehicle accidents. Heavy sleet is a relatively rare event, defined as an accumulation of ice pellets covering the ground to a depth of one-half-inch or more. Certain parts of the United States are known to have had episodes of heavy sleet.

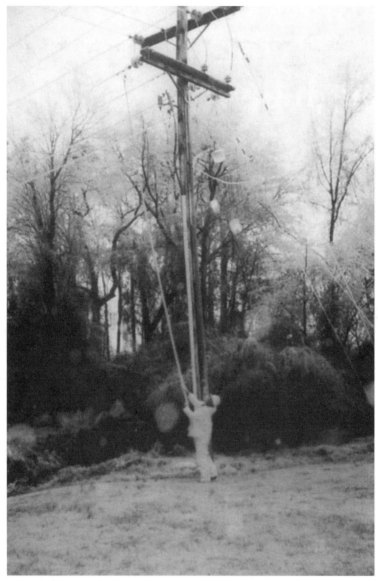

**Figure 4.4. A power company crew repairs downed wires.**

Ice and sleet storms generally occur from October through late April but these storms can sometimes happen into early May. The month of March has, for many areas of the country, on average, the greatest number of days in which freezing rain and freezing drizzle occurs, according to the National Weather Service (NWS).

The National Weather Service notes that more than 85 percent of all ice storm deaths are due to a traffic-related accident/event. Please keep in mind that as emergency managers we must often travel during these storms and, therefore, we are not immune to the hazards caused by these storms and their affects on the roads. A related statistic from the Occupational Safety and Health Administration is that the leading cause of workplace accidents, nationwide, is from motor vehicle accidents—that is a very startling bit of information, given all of the driving that emergency managers perform in a given year.

### Thunderstorms

Thunderstorms are the most common summer storm in most regions of the United States. These occur primarily during the months of May through August, with the most severe storms most likely to occur in the months of June and July.

Thunderstorms are usually localized and produced by cumulonimbus clouds. They are always accompanied by lightning and often have very strong wind gusts, heavy rain, and sometimes hail and tornadoes associated with them. Straight-line winds and heavy rain associated with thunderstorms are a great concern for many parts of the country.

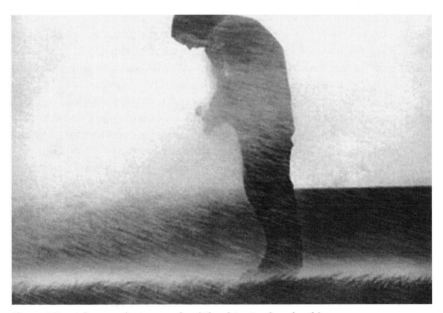

**Figure 4.5. A heavy rainstorm makes it hard to stand up for this emergency manager.**

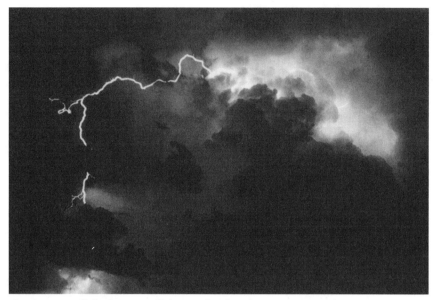

**Figure 4.6.   A lightning storm lights up the sky.**

## Lightning

Lightning is caused by the discharge of electricity between clouds or between clouds and the earth. In a thunderstorm, there is a rapid gathering of particles of moisture into the clouds and this activity results in the formation of large drops of rain. This gathering of moisture builds an electric potential until the surface of the cloud (or the enlarged water particles) is insufficient to carry the charge and a discharge takes place, producing a brilliant flash of light.

The power of the electrical charge and intense heat associated with lightning can electrocute a person on contact. It can also split trees, ignite fires, and cause electrical failures. The National Weather Service reports that most lightning casualties occur in the summer months, during the afternoon and early evening hours.

Lightning causes several wildfires per year nationwide, with the average annual suppression costs totaling millions of dollars; average annual damages also total millions of dollars.

## Tornadoes

Tornadoes are violently rotating columns of air rising up into a cloud. A thunderstorm is the first step in the creation of a tornado. A thunderstorm happens when there is moisture in the atmosphere; a lifting force causes air to begin ris-

**TABLE 4.1**
**Fujita Scale**

| | |
|---|---|
| F0: 40–72 MPH | F3: 158–206 MPH |
| F1: 73–112 MPH | F4: 207–260 MPH |
| F2: 113–157 MPH | F5: 261–318 MPH |

ing, and unstable air will continue to rise once it starts. Then, if other conditions are correct, the thunderstorm may spin out one or more tornadoes.

The Fujita scale rates the strength of a tornado. The wind speeds associated with each rating are listed in table 4.1.

## Hailstorms

Hailstorms are a product of severe thunderstorms. Hail is formed when strong updrafts within the storm carry water droplets above the freezing level, where they remain suspended and continue to grow larger, until their weight can no longer be supported by the winds. Hailstones can vary in size, depending on the strength of the updraft.

The National Weather Service (NWS) uses the descriptions in table 4.2 when estimating hail sizes.

Individuals who serve as volunteer "storm spotters" for the NWS are located throughout the country, and are instructed to report hail of dime size (three-fourths-inch) or greater. These spotters can be of great help to emergency managers with their reports.

Hailstorms can occur throughout the year; however, the months of maximum hailstorm frequency are typically between May and August. Although hailstorms rarely cause serious injury or loss of life, they can cause significant damage to property. Hailstorms are a common occurrence but damage is typically minimal and related to roofs, siding, and vehicles.

## Windstorms

Windstorms can and do occur in all months of the year, all across the country. However, the most severe windstorms usually occur during severe thunderstorms, which occur in the warm months of the summer.

**TABLE 4.2**
**Terms for hailstone sizes**

| | |
|---|---|
| Pea size is ¼-inch | Quarter size is 1-inch |
| Marble size is ½-inch | Golf ball size is 1¾-inches |
| Dime size is ¾-inch | Baseball size is 2¾-inches |

Some parts of the country have severe windstorms that are straight-line winds or downbursts associated with strong thunderstorms. A *downburst* is a severe localized downdraft from a thunderstorm or a rain shower. This outflow of cool or colder air can create damaging winds at or near the surface. The NWS reports indicate that winds up to 130 MPH have been recorded in some of the strongest thunderstorms. Often times, downburst winds can cause as much damage as a small tornado and are frequently confused with tornadoes because of the extensive damage that accompany them. As these downburst winds spread out, they are often referred to as straight-line winds. They can cause major structural and tree damage across a relatively large area. They can also create a hazard for small watercraft.

Winds of greater than 60 MPH are also associated with intense winter, spring, and fall low-pressure systems. These can also cause damage to buildings and in some cases overturn vehicles. This type of windstorm can impact residents living in coastal areas; winds can damage watercraft, waterfront homes, docks, and marinas.

Common items such as cans and bottles, signs, trees, glass, roof shingles, lawn furniture, and toys can become flying debris or projectiles in high winds. They frequently cause severe property damage, major injuries, and even death.

The extent of damage that a storm may cause is based on its wind speed. Table 4.3 shows wind speed and effects.

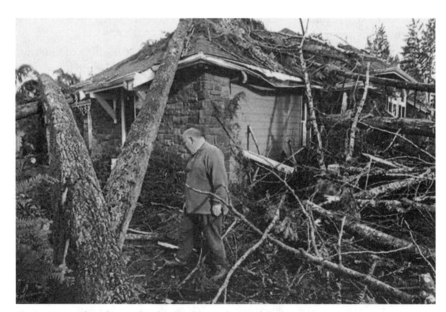

**Figure 4.7.   The aftermath of a windstorm in Washington State.**

**TABLE 4.3**
**The effects of wind at various speeds**

| Wind Speed (MPH) | Wind Effects |
|---|---|
| 25–31 | Movement of large branches. |
| 32–38 | Whole trees in motion; walking is difficult against the wind. |
| 39–54 | Small branches may break off trees; wind generally impedes progress when walking; trucks and motor homes may be difficult to control. |
| 55–74 | Potential damage to TV antennas; may push over shallow-rooted trees especially if the soil is drenched. |
| 74–95 | Potential for minor structural damage, especially to mobile homes; power lines, signs, and tree branches may be blown down. |
| 96–110 | Moderate structural damage to walls, roofs, and windows; large signs and tree branches blown down; moving vehicles blown off roads. |
| 111–130 | Extensive structural damage to walls, roofs, and windows; large trees blown down; mobile homes may be destroyed; vehicles destroyed. |
| 131–155 | Extreme damage to vehicles, structures and roofs; trees uprooted or snapped. |
| Greater than 155 | Catastrophic damage; structures destroyed. |

## Extreme Temperatures

### Summer Heat

Human beings need to maintain a constant body temperature if they are to stay healthy. Working in and being exposed to high temperatures induces heat stress when more heat is absorbed into the body than can be dissipated. Heat illness such as prickly heat, fainting from heat exhaustion, and heat cramps are visible signs that people are working in unbearable heat. In the most severe cases, the body temperature control system will break down altogether and the body temperature will rise rapidly. This is called heat stroke and can be fatal. The National Weather Service will issue a heat advisory when, during a twenty-four-hour period, the heat index ranges from 105 to 114 degrees Fahrenheit during the day and remains at or above 80 degrees F at night.

### Winter Cold

Winter can be an atrocious time. This is especially true and very dangerous for disabled citizens and any outdoor workers (including emergency management staff). Record temperature lows and arctic-like wind-chill factors can cause cold-related illness such as frostbite and hypothermia, which can be deadly. Hypothermia is the greatest and most life-threatening cold-weather danger.

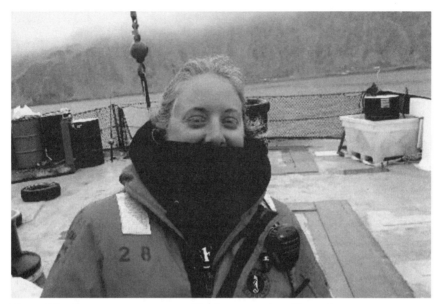

**Figure 4.8.   Emergency manager working in extremely cold weather.**

Hypothermia occurs when a person's core body temperature drops below 96 degrees F. Anyone who is exposed to severe cold without enough protection can develop hypothermia. Frostbite will occur when skin tissue and blood vessels are damaged from exposure to temperatures below 32 degrees F. Frostbite most commonly affects the extremities—toes, fingers, earlobes, chin, cheeks, nose, and other body parts that are often left uncovered in very cold temperatures. The National Weather Service issues a wind-chill warning when widespread wind chills of 60 degrees below zero or lower with winds greater than 10 MPH are expected.

## Flooding

Melting snow from heavy snows and rain from slow-moving thunderstorms and heavy downpours can cause localized flooding that can seriously impact property and infrastructure such as roads and bridges. Often this flooding is not related to structures being located in flood plains but is a result of stormwater management or limited capacity of the soil to absorb water due to frost in the ground, particularly in early spring, resulting in many flooded basements.

Besides snowmelt and heavy rains, a third type of flooding results from poor infrastructure (for example, inadequate sewer and stormwater management systems such as ditches, catch basins, and culverts). Finally, rising river, lake, and stream levels can cause flooding. This type of flooding is usually caused by

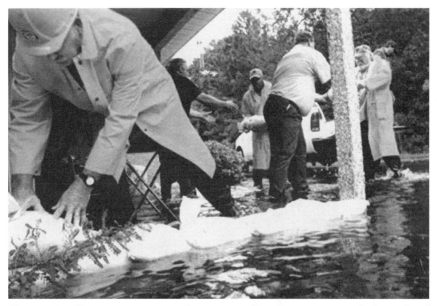

**Figure 4.9. These emergency workers are sandbagging a property during a flood situation.**

long-term, above-average precipitation with a poor outlet. Some other issues of flooding include:

- Flooding as a result of beaver dams is a concern in some rural areas of the United States.
- A number of flooded areas may not be mapped as floodplains on Flood Insurance Rate Maps from FEMA. Stormwater and runoff are the primary source of flooding waters in these areas.

## Drought

A drought refers to an extended period of deficient rainfall relative to the statistical mean for a region.

Drought can be defined according to meteorological, hydrological, socioeconomic, and agricultural criteria.

- Meteorological drought is qualified by any noteworthy shortfall of precipitation.
- Hydrological drought is apparent in noticeably reduced river and stream flow and critically low groundwater tables.

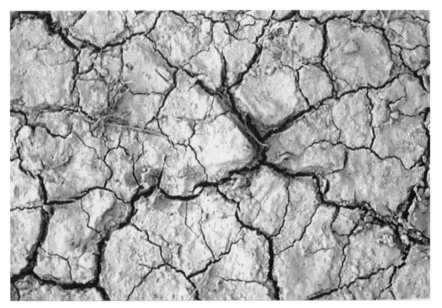

**Figure 4.10.  The ground in Florida during a period of drought.**

- Agricultural drought indicates an extended dry period that results in stress on crops and a reduction in harvest.
- Socioeconomic drought refers to the situation that occurs when water shortages begin to affect people and their lives. It associates economic goods with the elements of meteorological, agricultural, and hydrological drought. It is different from the other definitions because this drought type is based on the process of supply and demand. Many economic goods (such as water, food crops, fish, and hydroelectric power) have their supplies greatly dependent on the weather. Due to natural variations in climate, some years have high supplies of water and other years experience a low supply.

A socioeconomic drought takes place when the supply of an economic good cannot meet the demand for that product, and the cause of this shortfall is weather-related (water supply). Droughts in many areas of the country are of particular concern for emergency managers because of the high potential for forest fires coupled with the impacts lower lake/river levels have on the recreation industry.

## Wildfires

Wildfire is ranked as one of the greatest threats for emergency managers in many parts of the United States. The immediate danger from wildfires is the destruction of timber, property, and wildlife, as well as injury or loss of life to persons who live in the affected area or who are using recreational facilities in the area. Response personnel are also a big concern. Over the last several years, many firefighters have been seriously injured or killed in these fires.

Long-term effects from wildfires are numerous. Forest fires can leave large amounts of scorched and barren land that may not return to its pre-fire condition for many years. Major fires can completely destroy ground cover, which can, in turn, cause erosion and more damage to surrounding lands. As a result of population growth in rural forested areas, the potential for losses of life and property due to wildfires is greater now than in the past.

## Infectious Diseases

In the years immediately following World War II, many life-threatening infectious diseases were cured using antibiotics. Many diseases that couldn't be cured could be prevented through vaccinations. Currently, new diseases continue to emerge. New strains of influenza seem to rear their ugly heads on a yearly basis and require annual updates of vaccinations.

The recent introduction of diseases such as SARS and avian flu, for which scientists claim there is no cure or vaccination, as well as bioterrorism threats, highlight the need for a good public health system to detect new diseases early, in order to prevent a large-scale pandemic. The increased resistance of many diseases to various antibiotics available is another area of concern that emergency managers need to work together on with public health officials.

Another immediate concern surrounds diseases impacting livestock, including hoof and mouth disease that recently resurged in Europe is mad cow disease. Infectious disease outbreaks can easily occur as primary events themselves or they may be secondary events to another disaster or emergency, such as a terrorist attack or natural disaster.

## Earthquakes

An earthquake is defined as a shaking or trembling of the crust of the earth by underground volcanic forces or by breaking and shifting of rock underneath the surface.

Over time, stresses build beneath the earth's surface as part of its standard, ever-changing nature. From time to time, stress is released, which results in the sudden and often devastating shaking that we refer to as an earthquake. There is no warning system provided to us as to when an earthquake could occur; it can last for a few seconds or even longer. Larger earthquakes and their aftershocks can cause considerable damage to property, people, and infrastructure.

Fortunately, large earthquakes are not a common occurrence in most parts of the United States, but they do happen and have caused a great deal of damage, especially on the West Coast. As emergency managers, we cannot afford to be complacent because seismologists have indicated there is future potential for damaging earthquakes throughout the country, on both East and West Coasts.

As many of us know, earthquakes are one of the most costly natural hazards faced by the country. Earthquakes also pose a significant risk to approximately 75 million Americans in some thirty-nine states (which could experience an earthquake).

The risks that earthquakes pose to the public, including death, injury, and great economic loss, can be significantly reduced by:

- Better planning, building construction, and mitigation practices before earthquakes ever happen, and
- Providing critical and timely information to improve disaster response after they occur.

Table 4.4 shows the earthquake magnitude scale and the physical effects of earthquakes. Earthquakes are also classified in categories ranging from minor to great, depending on their magnitude, as seen in table 4.5.

**TABLE 4.4**
**Earthquake Magnitude Scale**

| Magnitude | Earthquake Effects |
|---|---|
| 2.5 or less | Usually not felt, but can be recorded by seismograph |
| 2.5 to 5.4 | Often felt, but only causes minor damage |
| 5.5 to 6.0 | Slight damage to buildings and other structures |
| 6.1 to 6.9 | May cause a lot of damage in very populated areas |
| 7.0 to 7.9 | Major earthquake; serious damage |
| 8.0 or greater | Enormous earthquake; may totally destroy communities near the epicenter |

**TABLE 4.5**
**Earthquake Magnitude Classes**

| Class | Magnitude |
|---|---|
| Great | 8 or more |
| Major | 7–7.9 |
| Strong | 6–6.9 |
| Moderate | 5–5.9 |
| Light | 4–4.9 |
| Minor | 3–3.9 |

## Summary

Every state in the United States can potentially experience the natural disasters that occur elsewhere in the world, especially those that have been described above. Some types of natural disasters have not occurred as frequently in some states as in other parts of the country or perhaps the world, but natural hazards can potentially be significant and very devastating.

# 5

# Technological Hazards and Terrorism

TECHNOLOGICAL HAZARDS ARE HAZARDS presented by man. Human-caused hazards are intentional, criminal, malicious uses of force and violence to perpetrate disasters against people or property. Often, they can be the result of *terrorism*—actions intended to intimidate or coerce a government or the civilian population to further political or social objectives—which can be either domestic or international, depending on the origin, base, and objectives of the terrorist organization. Technological hazards also can be acts of individuals carried out for personal reasons. Some examples include:

- Structural fires
- Hazardous materials
- Water supply contamination
- Wastewater system failure
- Dam failure
- Radiological
- Terrorism

## Structural Fires

Fire is a rapid oxidation and a persistent chemical reaction that releases heat and light. A fire can be categorized as both a natural and a technological hazard that can occur both outside and inside of a building.

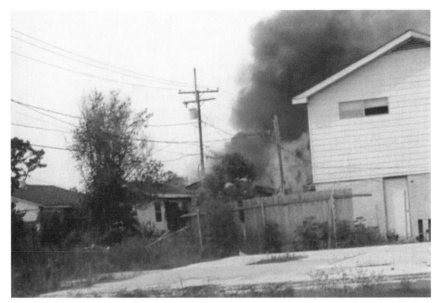

**Figure 5.1.   A structure fire in New Orleans.**

Structure fires are classified as:

- Residential
- Public/Mercantile
- Industrial/Manufacturing/Other Buildings

A second category of fires is vehicle fires, including:

- Aircraft
- Boats
- Trucks
- Busses
- Automobiles
- Trains

Cooking is the leading cause of home fires. It is also the leading cause of home fire injuries. Cooking fires often result from unattended cooking and human error, rather than mechanical failure of stoves or ovens.

Careless smoking is the leading cause of fire deaths. Smoke alarms and smolder-resistant bedding and upholstered furniture are significant fire deterrents. On July 8, 2006, Massachusetts approved Chapter 140 of the Acts of 2006, "An Act Relative to the Loss of Life Due to Fires Caused by Cigarettes." The new law is

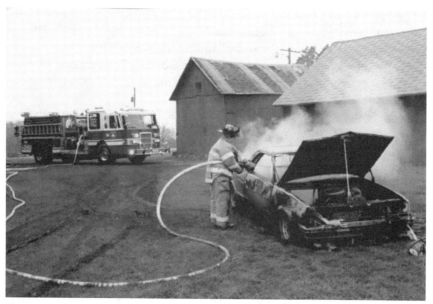

Figure 5.2.  A car on fire is a common sight in many communities.

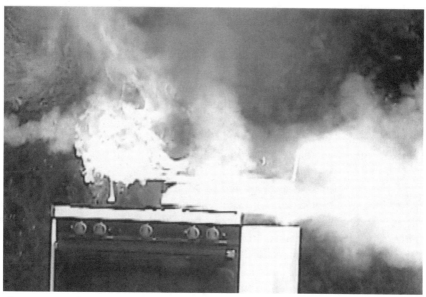

Figure 5.3.  A kitchen fire, caused by cooking, in a Massachusetts community.

now codified at M.G.L. c. 64C, § 2A-2F. The law requires that effective January 1, 2008, all cigarettes sold or offered for sale in Massachusetts shall meet the same testing criteria for fire-standard-compliant cigarettes as in New York State.

Arson is the second leading cause of both residential fires and residential fire deaths. In commercial properties, arson is the major cause of deaths, injuries, and financial loss.

Heating is the third leading cause of residential fires. Heating fires are a larger problem in single-family homes than in apartments. Unlike apartments, the heating systems in single-family homes are often not professionally maintained.

Emergency managers must work very closely with fire officials during any fire type of emergency, as these type of disasters may require evacuation, sheltering, and requests for additional resources.

## Hazardous Materials

Hazardous materials are made of substances that are flammable or combustible, that are explosive, toxic, lethal, or corrosive, or are oxidizers or radioactive. Business types that routinely use hazardous materials locally include the following:

- Hospitals
- Schools
- Metal plating shops
- Public utilities
- Fuel companies
- Communications companies
- Chemical distributors and manufacturers
- Research facilities/labs
- High technology firms
- Many others

Many of these businesses are required to develop and maintain plans for warning, notification, evacuation, and site security under various regulations. Hazardous materials incidents are generally associated with transportation related accidents or accidents at fixed facilities.

Hazardous materials may also be released as a secondary result of natural disasters such as large brush fires, hurricanes, and floods. In any case, buildings or vehicles can release their hazardous materials inventories rather quickly, when they are structurally compromised or are involved in transportation (vehicle) accidents. Pipelines can also be exposed or ruptured from collapsed embankments, vehicle accidents, road washouts, bridge collapses, and breaks in streets.

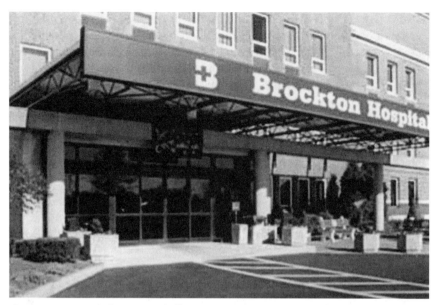

Figure 5.4.    Hospitals present challenges to emergency personnel.

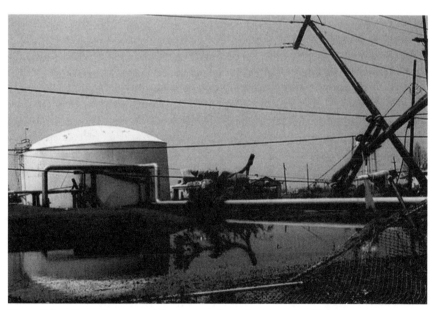

Figure 5.5.    Hazardous materials can be released as a result of hurricane damage.

Spills of hazardous materials might cause the short-term or long-term evacuation of an affected area. Depending on the nature of the spill and local weather conditions, the residences, businesses, hospitals, schools, nursing homes, and roadways in the area may be evacuated or closed to traffic until cleanup can be accomplished.

Emergency managers need not be trained as hazardous material technicians; however, it is extremely important that they have a thorough understanding of how these materials act and react with other materials, how the weather affects them, and what hazardous materials are located (and where) in their own community. Planning for a hazardous material event should be a priority.

Hazardous materials are transported throughout the country by road, rail, boat, air, and pipeline. Transported hazardous materials include materials moving from producers to users, moving between storage and use facilities, and hazardous waste moving from generators to treatment, storage, and disposal facilities (TSDF). Risks are obviously the greatest in the more populated areas along major transportation routes.

Many communities have an airport that serves the region for both pleasure and business flights. A variety of flammable liquids and chemicals are stored at these airports to be used for the airplanes and support vehicles. Accidents involving aircraft and chemicals related to their operation create a potential situation where hazardous materials could be released. In addition, the risk of an incident is further increased by any hazardous cargo that may be brought into the facility for transport.

## Water Supply Contamination

Water supply contamination can occur through the introduction of point and nonpoint source pollutants into public groundwater and/or surface water supplies. While water treatment systems in this country are very good and compromised public water supplies are rare, water contamination is still a concern.

Point source pollution comes from concentrated originating points like a pipe from a factory, although many other sources, including vehicles like tanker trucks and barges, have been legally interpreted to be point sources. Point sources are regulated by federal, state, and/or local laws and are required to have National Pollutant Discharge Elimination System (NPDES) permits from the appropriate state or federal EPA office.

Nonpoint source pollution is composed of pollutants from sources that are not required to have a NPDES permit. Nonpoint source pollution (NPS) concerns for communities include:

- Fertilizer runoff from both rural and urban areas
- Pesticide runoff from both rural and urban areas

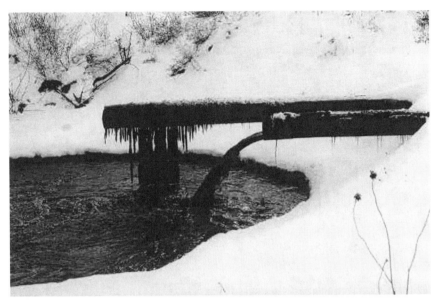

Figure 5.6.   This factory pipe is an example of point source pollution.

- Animal waste management
- Paint, oil, antifreeze, and other contaminants poured directly into storm drains
- Activities near a water source that can easily be contaminated without care
- Illegal dump sites
- Failing septic systems
- Soil erosion

The causes of water contamination are numerous and range from failing septic systems and leaking underground tanks to improper use of household chemicals. Many residences near lakes and rivers often have wells that use shallow groundwater that is particularly at risk for contamination. Seasonal homes or cottages in many areas of the country may have older wells that may need repair or replacement, but are a lower priority than the primary residence.

The most obvious concern about an unsafe water supply is the health risk to family or guests. Water contamination serves as a source of bacteria, viruses, and parasites that can cause gastrointestinal problems or transmit contagious diseases.

An emergency situation involving water contamination will require close communication by the emergency manager with the health agent, health inspector, or other health department official. These public health professionals have a great deal of knowledge in this area and can be helpful working toward a successful conclusion of the event.

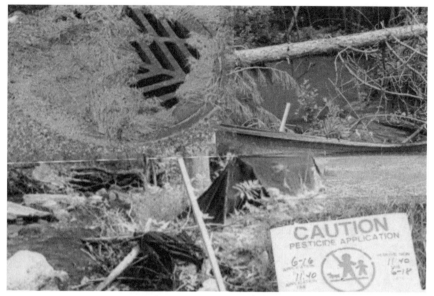

**Figure 5.7.   Pesticide runoff from farms is an example of nonpoint source pollution.**

## Wastewater System Failure

Wastewater collection systems often receive additional water during heavy storm events as a result of inflow and infiltration. This may cause the local wastewater treatment system to reach its maximum treatment capacity. In this event, excess flow will be directed into waterways untreated, resulting in sewage contamination. Inflow and infiltration is a problem for many communities as a result of aging infrastructure. Many communities have problems with their collecting systems causing severe sewer overflows.

Septic tanks are enclosures that store and process wastes where no sewer system exists. Septic tanks are especially prevalent in rural areas. Treatment of waste in septic tanks occurs by bacterial decomposition. The resulting material is called sludge. Contamination of water from septic tanks can occur under various conditions, including:

- Poor placement of septic leach fields (this can feed partially treated wastewater into a drinking water source). Leach fields are part of the septic system for land-based tanks and include an area where wastewater percolates through soil as part of the treatment process.
- Badly constructed percolation systems may allow water to escape without proper treatment.
- System failure can result in clogging and overflow to land or surface water.

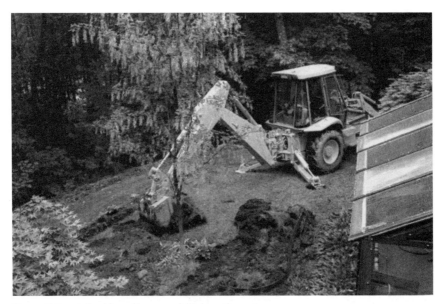

Figure 5.8. A backhoe digs up a failed septic system.

High-density placement of tanks, such as in suburban areas, can result in regions containing very high concentrations of wastewater. This water may seep to the land surface, run off into surface water, or flow directly into the water table.

Emergency managers must work closely with the local department of public works, water or sewer department, and health department in the event of wastewater contamination. These events can also cause the transmittal of contagious diseases and gastrointestinal illnesses. Many communities have instituted an educational program for residents to outline some of the hazards of failed systems and the other issues mentioned above.

## Dam Failure

Dam failures can result in major flooding and severe damage to property and loss of life. There have been several dam failures in the United States that have resulted in major damages or loss of life, according to the Federal Energy Regulatory Commission (FERC). Dams can also cause problems when they are not managed and operated properly. A problem at a dam would most likely occur during a flood event but could occur anytime.

Dam safety is regulated at the state and federal level. Some states have a number of hydro dams for electricity production and headwaters dams for storage of water for hydropower production. The dams that are part of hydropower

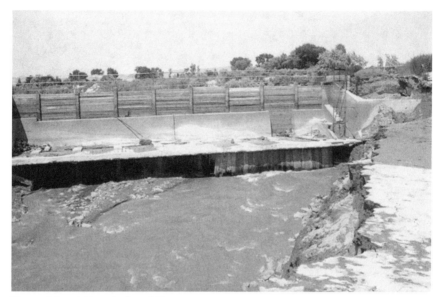

**Figure 5.9. A Nevada dam failure.**

production are regulated through the FERC. Nonfederal dams are under the regulatory jurisdiction of the various states involved or, perhaps, the U.S. Army Corps of Engineers.

Many residences in neighborhoods near dams would be severely impacted if a hydro facility failed. Dams upstream from a facility could cause a cascading effect if there was ever a malfunction.

The Federal Emergency Management Agency (FEMA) has a National Dam Safety Program. This program is intended to help states bring the necessary resources to bear on inspection, classification, and emergency planning with respect to dam safety.

The National Inventory of Dams (NID) is a computer database used to track information on the nation's water control infrastructure. Information from the NID is used in the development of water resource management, land use management, flood plain management, risk management, and emergency action planning.

FERC regulates and licenses nonfederally owned hydroelectric dams that are exempt from state rules and regulations. These facilities are required to have an emergency plan in place identifying the areas that could be impacted and the response in case of a dam failure.

## Radiological Hazards

A radiological hazard is the potential for exposure to materials that emit ionizing radiation. The primary radiological danger is the health effects resulting from

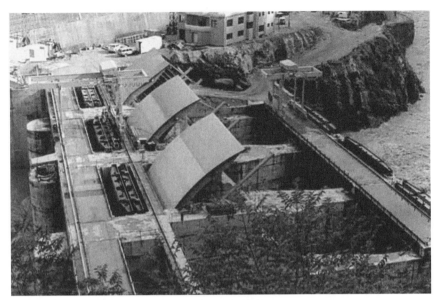

**Figure 5.10.   A large, operating hydroelectric dam.**

unintentional exposure. When radiation interacts with atoms, energy is deposited, resulting in ionization (electron excitation). This ionization could damage certain critical molecules or structures in cells. Ionizing radiation is emitted from molecular elements generally referred to as radionuclides. This radiation also has the ability to alter, in varying amounts, the function of living processes at the cellular level. Types of ionizing radiation include:

- Alpha particles
- Beta particles
- Gamma rays
- X-rays
- Neutron particles

Radiation is measured in different ways. Measurements used in the United States include Roentgen, radiation absorbed dose (RAD), and roentgen equivalent man (REM). The term *RAD* is being replaced by the international system unit for radiation absorbed dose, the gray (Gy), which is a measurement of absorbed dose in any material; 1 Gy = 100 RAD.

The nature and extent of damage caused by ionizing radiation depend on a number of factors, including the amount of exposure (energy strength), the frequency and/or duration of exposure, and the penetrating power of the radiation to which an individual is exposed. Acute exposure to very high doses of ionizing radiation is rare but can cause death within a few days or months. The sensitivity of the exposed cells also influences the extent of damage. For example, rapidly

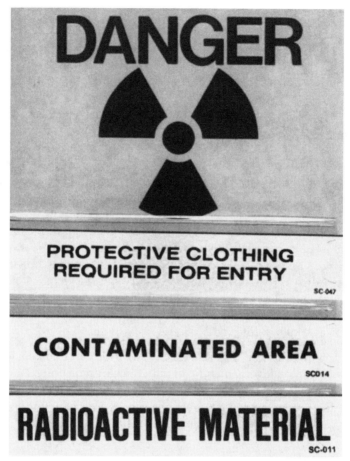

DANGER

PROTECTIVE CLOTHING
REQUIRED FOR ENTRY

SC-047

CONTAMINATED AREA

SC014

RADIOACTIVE MATERIAL

SC-011

**Figure 5.11.   A radiation sign indicates a potential hazard.**

growing tissues, such as developing embryos, are particularly vulnerable to harm from ionizing radiation.

Nuclear power plants are a significant potential source of ionizing radiation. The health and environmental impacts from the Three-Mile Island (Pennsylvania) and Chernobyl (Russia) disasters demonstrate the potential hazards from nuclear power plants. In communities that have a nuclear plant, the emergency manager will need to interact with the plant officials regarding emergency planning issues and other important topics. Other sources of ionizing radiation include medical and diagnostic X-ray machines, certain surveying instruments, some imaging systems used to check pipelines, and radioactive sources used to calibrate radiation detection instruments.

On December 7, 1979, following the Three Mile Island nuclear power plant accident in March of that year, President Carter transferred the federal lead role in offsite radiological emergency planning and preparedness activities from the

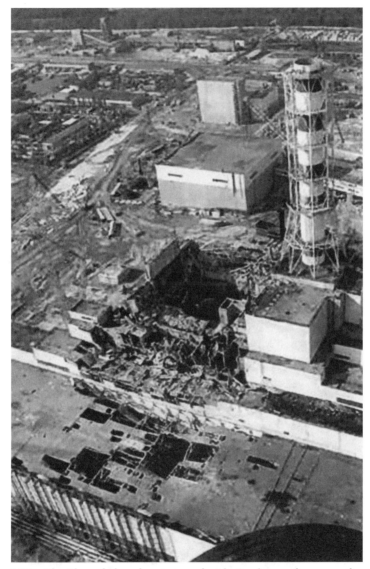

**Figure 5.12.   The Chernobyl nuclear power plant in Russia was the scene of a serious radiation accident.**

Nuclear Regulatory Commission (NRC) to the Federal Emergency Management Agency (FEMA). FEMA then established the Radiological Emergency Preparedness (REP) program to:

- Ensure that the public health and safety of citizens living around commercial nuclear power plants would be adequately protected in the event of a nuclear power station accident, and

- Inform and educate the public about radiological emergency preparedness. FEMA's REP program responsibilities encompass only "offsite" activities— that is, state and local government emergency preparedness activities that take place beyond the nuclear power plant boundaries. Onsite activities continue to be the responsibility of the Nuclear Regulatory Commission.

University laboratories, medical treatment facilities, medical laboratories, hospitals, clinics, and doctor's offices also contain a large number of radionuclides. These materials are used in research, diagnostics, and treatment. Emergency managers should have an idea of what locations in their communities have or use radionuclides.

At the federal and national levels, there are a number of agencies/groups that have capabilities to respond to radiological emergencies. These include:

- U.S. Department of Energy (DOE)
- Nuclear Regulatory Commission (NRC)
- Federal Emergency Management Agency (FEMA)
- U.S. Department of Transportation (DOT)
- American Nuclear Society (ANS)

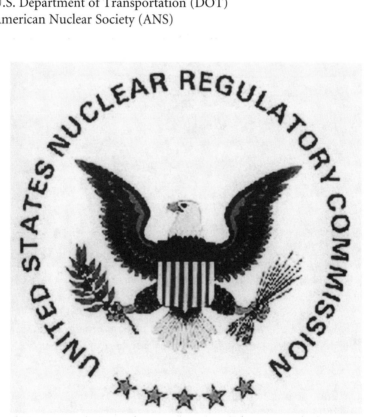

Figure 5.13.   The Nuclear Regulatory Commission (NRC) logo.

State hazardous materials (hazmat) teams also have equipment to respond to a radiological incident. The Federal Radiological Emergency Response Plan (FRERP) is in place to establish an organized and integrated capability for a timely, coordinated response by federal agencies to peacetime radiological emergencies.

## Terrorism

Several threats can result from terrorist activity. Terrorist activities that could occur in most communities include:

- Biological
- Chemical
- Nuclear
- Radiological
- Arson
- Incendiary
- Explosives
- Armed attacks
- Industrial sabotage
- Intentional hazardous materials releases
- Cyberterrorism

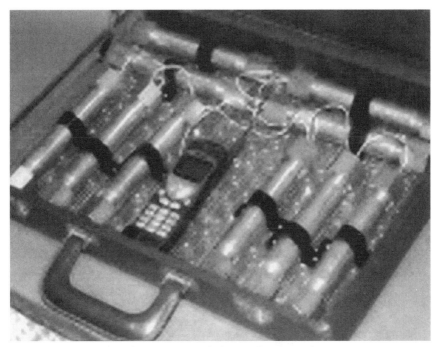

Figure 5.14. A suitcase bomb using explosives and a phone detonator.

Several places in your community could be potential targets for terrorism. What places are you thinking about while reading this section? Do you have an airport, hospital, stadium, arena, courthouse, power plant, or port? Did you think about all the school buildings in your community and the violent incidents that have occurred in schools over the last several years? There are other potential targets, such as power and pipeline infrastructure, and roadway infrastructure such as bridges and tunnels. Emergency managers need to be aware of these potential targets and have plans in place to deal with possible terrorist activity. They should also maintain current contact information for officials in charge of these facilities.

The Coast Guard is responsible for conducting a risk assessment for facilities in the country's ports or waterfront areas as part of their Maritime Security Plan. Just as I have encouraged cooperation with officials involved in other technological hazards, in areas where the Coast Guard operates, the emergency manager needs to be in communication with the harbormaster, local Coast Guard officials, and, of course, the law enforcement community. All of us need to share information regarding terrorism, including threats and occurrences of suspicious individuals, packages, and vehicles.

The strategy of many terrorists is to achieve acts of aggression that attract the attention of people in the community, the government (federal, state, and local), and the world to their particular cause. The terrorists plan their attacks to obtain the greatest amount of publicity they can possibly garner, often selecting targets that stand for exactly what they are against. How effective the terrorists will be depends partially upon what they decide to do and in the emergency management's response to the terrorist act.

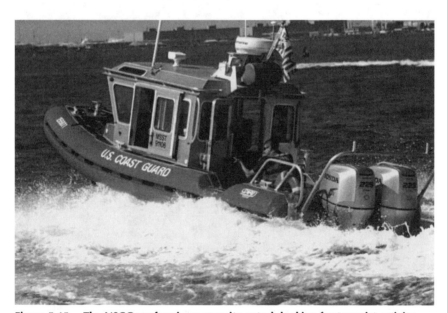

**Figure 5.15.   The USCG performing a security patrol, looking for terrorist activity.**

# 6

# How to Manage Volunteers

W HEN A DISASTER STRIKES, regardless of the location, most people's natural tendency is to offer some type of assistance. Most of us are taught as youngsters to help our neighbors, relatives, and other people in times of need. Often, people flock to the scene of a disaster and want to help in whatever capacity may be needed, not realizing that they can be in the way. Responding to the scene without being called (called self-deployment) can create a "disaster" within the disaster. This can also cause traffic problems, issues for law enforcement agencies and other emergency agencies responding to and dealing with the incident, and a host of other probable and possible troubles. Just think about how many issues you can think of, now, that may be caused by people "just showing up" at a disaster scene!

Many emergency situations, especially a large-scale crisis, can benefit from the use of volunteers. How the volunteer helpers are dealt with can make or break that portion of the disaster response. The use of volunteers is not always encouraged or warranted; however, if volunteers are needed, there is a definite place for them, provided they are managed properly. The fact that volunteers are not always encouraged to participate in an emergency needs some explanation. Let me try to do that.

There are some emergencies, such as those involving criminal or terrorist activities, hazardous materials, or other situations where responders need very specific training. In these instances, it would not be wise to use volunteers in certain roles. There certainly is a great deal of liability involved, not to mention the potential to have the volunteers become victims themselves.

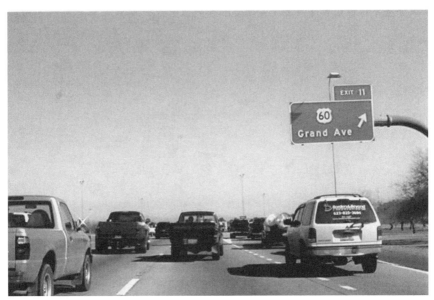

Figure 6.1.   A traffic jam.

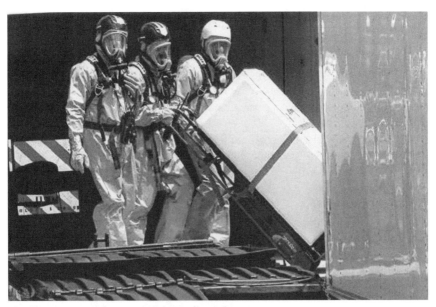

Figure 6.2.   Hazardous material team in action.

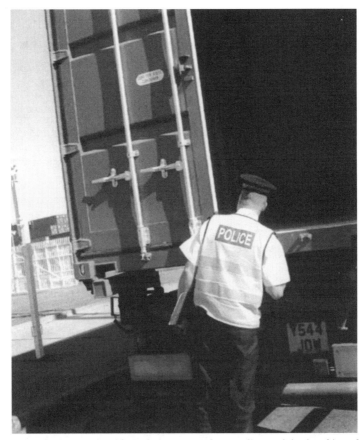

Figure 6.3.  **Volunteers should not be present where police activity is taking place.**

## The Professionals

In large-scale events, the police, fire, municipal administration, emergency medical, highway department, and emergency management officials (as well as others) within your community are initially going to be overwhelmed dealing with their "usual" response duties, as well as those related to the emergency. These "usual" duties can include the following:

- Evacuation
- Sheltering
- Traffic control
- Fire response
- Alarm sounding

- Lack of power
- Crime scene processing
- Motor vehicle accidents
- Other law enforcement issues
- Hazardous material response (spills, leaks and releases)
- Wires down
- Dealing with limbs and trees blocking roads
- Medical response to injured and ill residents and transients and guests
- Declaration of disaster
- Day-to-day administrative functions and duties

The professionals, during a disaster, will be inundated with calls from the public requesting information on what happened or what is happening. They may be reporting situations that require attention (some may be more serious than others). Some callers may also ask, "do you need help?" Other individuals may just feel like helping and show up at or near the scene or respond to the police department, fire station, or sheriff's office. (I can recall a situation where a large disaster was in progress and a resident called to ask if his help was needed and was told no. He then responded anyway to the scene with his station wagon, because he heard over the scanner that additional ambulances were needed and thought he could help instead of having the injured wait for ambulances.)

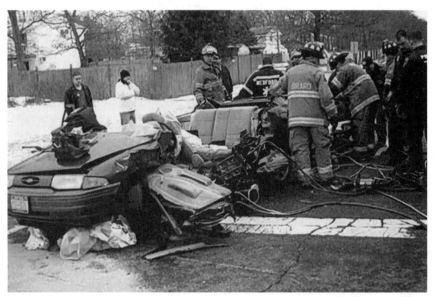

**Figure 6.4. A motor vehicle accident is a routine part of the day for some first responders.**

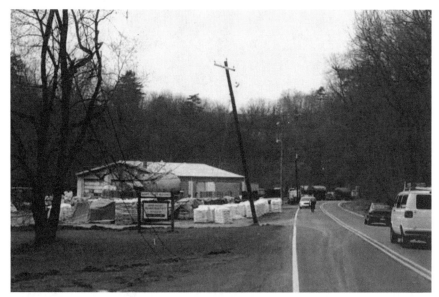

Figure 6.5.   Wires down always cause a problem.

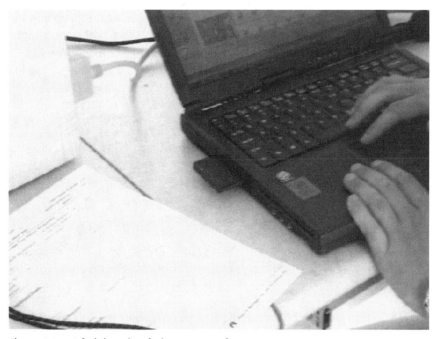

Figure 6.6.   Administrative duties must get done.

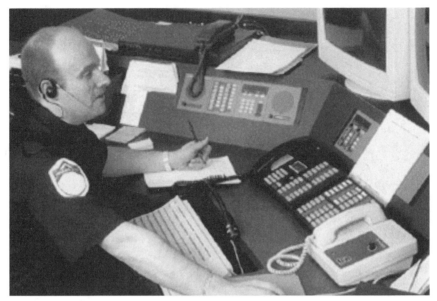

**Figure 6.7.   A dispatcher sends units in response to a call.**

Initially, the dispatchers may not have enough time or information to provide to these callers and, as a result, a large number of people want to help and have no direction, guidance, or leadership and can cause more problems by acting without authority, training, or direction.


## A Plan of Attack

It is always wise to have a plan of attack in place to deal with the onslaught of spontaneous volunteers and folks that want to help. Some thoughts should include the following:

- Location to direct volunteers for reporting, if needed
- Pre-determined idea of what to use volunteers for
- Pre-printed applications
- Supplies to deal with the application process (pens, paper, clipboards)
- If outdoors, a shelter (tent) to keep people out of the elements
- Water

A recent event following Hurricane Katrina put a Massachusetts sheriff's office in this position. Hundreds of people from at least three states showed up in an effort to help with evacuees that were due to arrive from Louisiana and Mississippi. The question became "Now what do we do with these volunteers?" The sheriff did not want to discourage people from helping, but there was no plan or procedure in place to deal with the large numbers of people, all showing up to help at the same time!

Within thirty minutes, they had a makeshift system in place to take applications. The applications were printed forms to gather much needed information, such as:

- Name, address, and contact information
- Any specialized training (nurse, teacher, physician, social worker)
- References
- Educational experience
- Employment history
- Availability

Some of this information eliminates these concerns:

- What can I do?
- I don't want to do that!

By having an application, the volunteer can tell you in what areas he/she does or does not want to help. It's never a good thing to have a volunteer assigned to a task they don't want to perform. Just imagine being assigned a task you don't want to perform in your own job—and then being a volunteer! There is no way you will ever get this person to volunteer again, if he/she is assigned a duty that is uncomfortable or difficult for them to perform. (See appendix G for a sample volunteer application.)

Additionally, the sheriff's personnel had the entire group fill out CORI (Criminal Offender Registry Information) forms. It was felt that this was extremely important to determine if any of the volunteers had criminal records—or worse, had outstanding warrants. Most of the group filled out the forms with no problem. However, a few actually said, "Thanks, but I don't think I want to fill out a CORI." They sat for a few minutes and then left quietly, so as to not to draw attention to themselves. Others, some with serious, prior criminal records, filled out the forms and had to be told that their services were not going to be needed. (Obviously, this should be done discreetly.) Some individuals that had minor criminal records were interviewed and at the discretion of a sheriff's office representative, they were allowed to stay or not. None of the volunteers had outstanding warrants, so no arrests had to be made!

In this case, filling out the CORI form and background check was important, as officials thought there was a potential for the volunteers to be exposed to children and others, so they didn't want someone with a violent past or a sexual

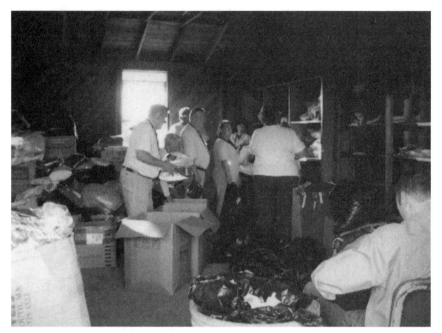

**Figure 6.8.   Volunteers in action.**

offender dealing with any of the evacuees. (Perhaps your group may also consider a sex offender registry check, in the event of a spontaneous volunteer opportunity in your community.) Once the background checks were conducted, a photo identification card indicating that the person was a volunteer was issued to any unpaid helper. This helped to alleviate some of the many daily checks that would be normally required by security officials and others.

Please keep in mind that not everyone is comfortable with all of the tasks that may be involved in the disaster operation. Remember, also, that they are volunteers, and you cannot force anyone to do a job! If a volunteer balks at performing a task that is assigned, reassign him/her to another job and get someone to replace him/her.

## Supervision

The emergency manager or other person in charge of the volunteers needs to direct the volunteers and keep them focused and involved. It is extremely important to thank every volunteer—every day! This is not too much to expect from the leadership, especially for people who don't have to be there. Remember, they are volunteers; they aren't getting paid. If they need to leave early or can't stay late, please don't yell or complain. Instead, thank them for their efforts and attempt to get another volunteer who can help with the work or project. Don't forget to say thank you!

Some of the other issues that come up for many emergency managers include the following:

- Food, water, breaks, sun block
- Daily safety briefings (reminders to people)
- Scheduling of volunteers for their work shift
- Tracking of personnel; monitoring sign in/out daily
- Documentation issues, who was present, what did they do, man-hours
- Lessons learned
- Let people know what is happening (keep them informed)
- Don't let them overstep their level of training or their roles and responsibilities
- Communication with volunteers should be within that group—volunteers should not be dealing with the incident command staff of the overall incident
- Don't let the volunteers get "too involved" dealing with the victims—they can become overwhelmed and perhaps be taken advantage of

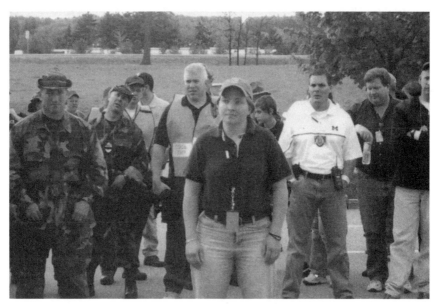

**Figure 6.9.   A safety briefing is a vital part of any operation.**

## Some Guidance

Please try to never let a volunteer's position interfere with his or her full-time job or family life. Tell the volunteers that "If you can be here, great!" Oftentimes, volunteers see the need for their assistance and they become caught up in the moment. Many times, they don't eat properly, as "they are too busy" helping. Also, their normal commitments to their family and work seem to be put on the back burner, because "they need me to be here." Volunteers should be told that they are appreciated; however, family and work should be priorities. I recall a particular couple who volunteered numerous hours. They were great workers and were extremely dedicated to their volunteerism. Some months later, I learned that they were so wrapped up in volunteering that they had forgotten family birthdays and her parents' anniversary. It needs to be stressed that as volunteers, their own lives come first. It is much better to be able to tend your own needs and those of your family and friends first, and then help the community.

## Buddy System

No volunteer should ever be allowed to work alone. Always try to stress the buddy system. It doesn't mean that they have to hold hands but it does mean they need to work as a team. The buddy system does many things for us:

- Two heads are better than one—usually!
- If someone needs help, the buddy will hopefully be able to call for assistance.
- Working with a buddy makes tasks easier, such as lifting.
- It gives people a chance to communicate with someone.

## Stress

Last but not least, I want to mention that dealing with a disaster or any type of emergency is a stressful situation. This goes for the professional but more so for the volunteer. Oftentimes the professionals have a system in place to deal with issues (such as an employee assistance program or critical incident stress counseling), whereas volunteers usually do not. Someone should be assigned to monitor the group of volunteers to ensure that they are:

- Not getting too involved
- Taking care of their personal needs
- Not becoming overwhelmed
- Dealing with the stress they are under because of involvement in the disaster

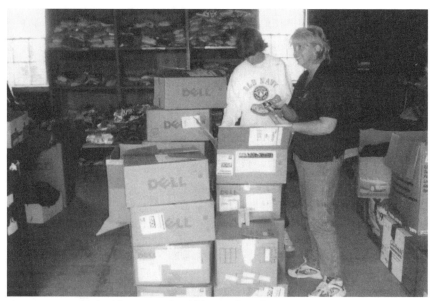

Figure 6.10.   The buddy system should be used at all times.

## Assigning Tasks and Planning to Manage Volunteers

Many volunteers may be needed to help respond to and recover from a major disaster. Volunteers can help more effectively if they have joined a group of people who have been trained for disaster work long before a disaster hits.

Disaster volunteers are able to perform a wide variety of tasks. Some examples of the jobs involved are:

- Administrative duties, such as telephone calls, filing, and documentation efforts
- Sheltering victims
- Meal preparations and feeding victims
- Medical triage/minor first-aid duties
- Sandbagging and heavy lifting
- Assessing property damage
- Ham radio or other communications
- Driving
- Delivery of goods to shut-ins and others
- Warehousing of supplies (disaster supplies)
- Light search techniques (missing or lost individuals)
- Coordinating other volunteers
- Cleanup
- Babysitting (for example, at shelters)

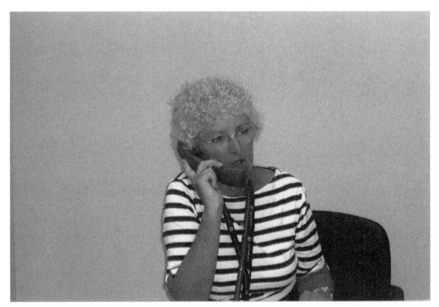

Figure 6.11.   Answering phones is not glamorous, but it has to be done.

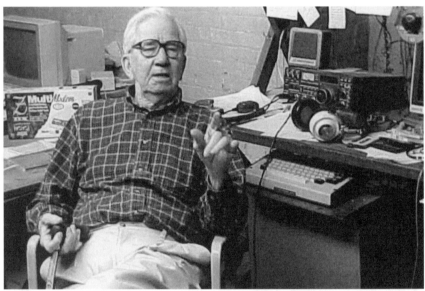

Figure 6.12.   Ham radio operators are an important part of many disasters for communications.

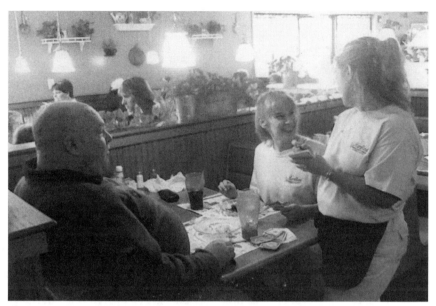

**Figure 6.13. My favorite restaurant, Marshland Too. Volunteers may be fortunate to get a good meal during times of disaster.**

No one job is any more important than the rest when so many things need to be done. The work is not always a glamorous assignment. In fact, most of the time, it is a lousy job that the volunteer is assigned. He may spend long, stressful days in less-than-ideal conditions. Overnight stays may be on cots (or the floor) in a school gymnasium. They may miss meals and the food that they do get may not be from their favorite restaurant or even meet their expectations.

But as difficult as the work may be, disaster volunteers consistently tell me that they have received more than they've given when they show up to help.

Emergency managers should prepare for the next disaster immediately. They should be thinking that in order to get help during the next disaster; these are some things to think about now:

- What skills are needed?
- Where can you get the training needed for some people to perform certain tasks? (Contact recognized disaster response agencies in your area to find out about training)
- What skills can people in your community contribute?
- What tasks are they interested in doing?
- Can your volunteers help out during their normal work time? (Many employers won't allow them to volunteer during work hours.)

When volunteers have matched their interests and skills with the jobs that may need to be done, they should register with a recognized disaster response agency in your area.

## Responding to Disasters

Many volunteers just show up to help at the time a large disaster strikes. Here are a few things to have the volunteers keep in mind when they show up during this first response phase:

- If you haven't been called to respond—Stop—and then call the group you've joined to find out if and where your help is needed, then arrange transportation to the site.
- Anticipate other needs. Do you need to bring food, water, extra clothes (socks), or a sleeping bag for an overnight stay in the disaster area? Will you need shovels, office supplies, or other tools for the tasks you'll be doing?
- Remember that you are priority number one. Protect your health and safety. Respond only if you are in shape for the tasks you'll be doing. Always be cautious about traveling in the dangerous weather that may accompany the disaster incident.
- Dress appropriately for the weather and for the tasks you'll be expected to perform.
- Affiliate before showing up. Instead of arriving unexpectedly in a disaster area, volunteers should register with a recognized volunteer agency. Also, do not self-deploy. Your group will call you if they need you or your skill set.
- Prepare for self-sufficiency. In most disasters, there are inadequate facilities for feeding, housing, personal hygiene, and health/medical needs for volunteers. It is best to affiliate with a recognized agency that will provide for these needs. However, it is always good to be prepared, just in case.
- Be patient and flexible. Volunteers should be prepared to step into any of a variety of roles, depending on current or sudden needs. Volunteers expecting to enter a response or relief effort in a certain capacity will often be disappointed. Sometimes a volunteer's unique talents are not immediately needed. They should also be advised to inform the supervisor or emergency manager if they are assigned to a task that they cannot physically or mentally perform.
- Know the liability situation. A volunteer should be certain that there is coverage by liability clauses in the insurance structure of the volunteer agency with which he or she is affiliated. A volunteer not registered with a volunteer agency should assume that all liability is entirely with the volunteer as an individual. Emergency managers should make this perfectly clear and perhaps even put it in writing for the volunteers.

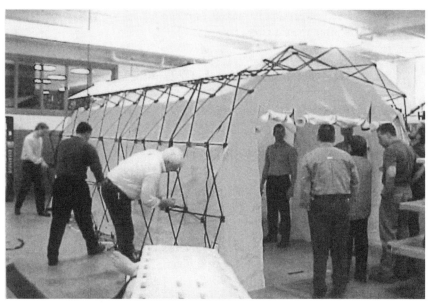

**Figure 6.14.   Volunteers perform a variety of tasks.**

- A coordinated process. The use of volunteers should be an organized process by which people with abilities, skills, and/or training are assigned to special tasks. Volunteers are most useful when they are able to do the right thing at the right time.
- Commit to the response effort. Disaster work is often dirty, monotonous, mundane, and not very glamorous. There is little, if any, individual recognition. As a result, some people won't become involved, and the volunteer should be prepared to accept this. Volunteers need to be committed to work under such conditions and fit within plans that are coordinated by their volunteer organization.

## Assistance in the Recovery Operations

A little-known fact is that it may take several years for disaster victims to put their lives back together. Volunteers are a very important part of this recovery process as they organize to help in stricken communities.

Immediate area cleanup is one task that may be needed shortly after the first response to the disaster. This can require a massive effort by many volunteers who show up to help. Some long-term recovery work will likely require volunteers with special skills or licenses. Two examples of such tasks are crisis counseling and rebuilding of damaged homes and businesses. Both of these tasks are critical after the disaster.

## Related Statues Regarding Protections for Volunteers

### 42 U.S.C. 14501 et seq. Volunteer Protection Act

This law preempts state laws to limit the liability of persons serving as volunteers for governmental and nonprofit organizations.

### State Laws

There may be individual state laws and local ordinances and bylaws that also pertain to the volunteer. Emergency managers should check with their state emergency management agency and their local governing body to see if there is additional coverage for the volunteer responders.

## Training

It is always recommended that volunteers receive training prior to the disaster. I would strongly recommend that they receive Incident Command System (ICS) training and NIMS training. Some other training courses are listed below.

- ICS 100—Introduction to the Incident Command System
- ICS 200—ICS for Single Resources and Initial Action Incidents
- IS 700—National Incident Management System (NIMS)
- IS 800—National Response Plan (just changed to the National Response Framework or NRF)

Another training program to consider would be a program put together for the emergency management staff. I would suggest a custom course that is designed to improve the participants' abilities to deal with the wide range of issues that result from managing volunteers. This course should address:

- Identification of tasks that require volunteer services
- Skill definition and specification of qualifications
- Publicity and recruitment
- Skill development and maintenance
- Disaster psychology
- Motivation strategy that promotes continued involvement
- Quality performance use of volunteers during a disaster
- Reviewing volunteer programs for effectiveness

## Who Is Going to Do All of This?

Many emergency managers have a staff that can assist with volunteer coordination. Believe me when I tell you that volunteer coordination is a full-time job in a disaster. The following is offered as an aid to emergency managers who might want to recruit a person to help in this effort.

## Job Descriptions

### Spontaneous Volunteer Coordinator

- Establish spontaneous volunteer reporting location at a designated location.
- Coordinate with various participating agencies to determine what training is needed and the experience levels of needed volunteers. Document opportunities for training, work performed, and so on.
- Process and direct the fulfillment of all volunteer requests.
- Establish and clearly communicate job assignments, rules, and volunteer code of conduct.
- Consult with and act as a technical resource to volunteer supervisors regarding potential personnel problems.
- Investigate complaints or problems and manage other personal action involving volunteers assigned through the spontaneous volunteer center.
- Oversee the Volunteer Screener.

### Volunteer Screener

- Ensure individuals processed through the spontaneous volunteer center undergo a consistent, nondiscriminatory screening procedure including an application, background check, and interview. They should receive proper identification.
- Start and maintain a master filing system. Engage and supervise additional volunteer screeners as needed.
- Work with spontaneous volunteer coordinator to fulfill volunteer requests.
- Arrange for the proper follow-up and thanking of volunteers assigned through the spontaneous volunteer center.
- Ensure proper disposition of volunteer records and files after operation.

## Summary

Adequate systems and processes have to be established by emergency managers before the disaster for referrals, screening, training, placement, and mobilization.

Without a process and a system in place, putting a large group of volunteers into an affected area with a compromised infrastructure, very limited resources, potential danger, and an emotionally charged atmosphere will strain any organization or agency. On top of this, without a plan in place, the professional emergency responders will have to be diverted to deal with the influx of volunteer responders.

The simple reality is that organizations that provide ways to prepare for and respond to disasters have an opportunity to build reputations, draw new volunteers, and develop new partnerships with other disaster-related groups.

There will always be spontaneous volunteers. There will always be people who will self-deploy. How you deal with these volunteers may well affect the next emergency in your jurisdiction.

# 7

# Pets and Emergencies

T HE ONLY WAY WE CAN REDUCE the devastation of a disaster like a hurricane is to be prepared. The more we prepare, the better our chances of reducing suffering and risk for our communities. One of the lessons learned from recent disasters is that we have not prepared very well for dealing with pets during emergencies.

## Expect the Unexpected

This phrase is repeated so often that it has almost lost its power and meaning. Does anyone really expect, never mind plan for, that one day his or her home, vehicle, possessions, and all means of communication will suddenly be gone? And, really, do people expect to find themselves in the same position as the unfortunate families that we saw on the news during the last winter storm, or flood, or fire?

Yet that's exactly what happens to many pet owners every year during these types of emergency situations. No matter where you live, the unexpected can occur. Disasters come in all forms. From blizzards to wildfires, earthquakes to hurricanes, terrorist attacks to floods, emergencies occur in all parts of the country, which means that everyone should have a disaster plan for their family—including a plan for pets.

## Planning for Anything

Remember that good disaster planning needs to take every possibility into consideration. For example, traffic accidents involving hazardous trucks can close streets and neighborhoods many miles away. What will you do if you are unable to get home to care for your pet? Make plans ahead of time. Arrange for a trusted neighbor who is frequently at home to evacuate your pets if an evacuation order is issued and you are at work. Keep a three-day supply of your pet's food, medicines, leash, veterinary records, and other necessities together in a pet carrier that is ready to go.

Many disasters occur without warning. However, if advance notice is given—whether it's two days or two hours—always take the necessary precautions. I recommend that people err on the safe side when it comes to their animals' care and their own safety. During many emergency situations, I've seen pet owners on television say that they waited far too long to get out of the area and, by the time the storm had arrived, they couldn't find their animals.

In the case of a severe weather alert, pet owners should put a piece of duct tape on their animal's collar with the name and number of a friend or relative living out of state since disasters can wipe out landlines and cell phone service for several days. So many more animals could potentially be saved if people would realize that all forms of communication can completely shut down indefinitely, making it nearly impossible for people to contact them, so any little thing they can do to help is great.

Horse owners/caretakers are equally susceptible to disasters, particularly barn fires. A new booklet from the Humane Society of the United States, *Making Your Horse Barn Fire Safe*, will help horse owners prevent tragedy and protect their horses and barns from fire-related injury and damage.

Here are some interesting facts from the American Pet Product Manufacturers Association (www.appma.org):

- There are approximately 65 million owned dogs in the United States.
- About 39 percent of U.S. households (or 40.6 million) own at least one dog.
- About 65 percent of owners have one dog, 23 percent have two dogs, and 12 percent have three or more dogs.
- There are approximately 77.6 million owned cats in the United States.
- About 34 percent of U.S. households (or 35.4 million) own at least one cat.
- About 51 percent of owners have one cat; the rest have two or more.

As emergency managers, we need to get the word out that if you live in or along any coastal area you must plan for hurricanes, and that planning should include your pets. Any disaster that threatens humans threatens animals as well. We have always told people that pets are not allowed in the shelters. This is not your father's Civil Defense anymore! Times have changed and some shelters are now allowing pets because people were refusing to be evacuated without their animals, often leading to other emergency situations and even deaths of pets and owners.

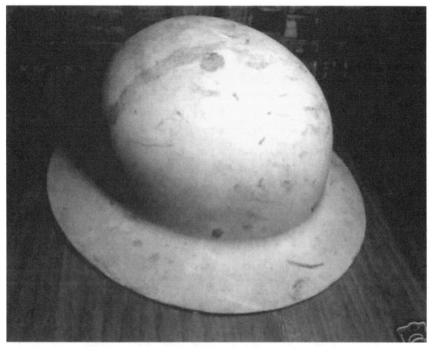

Figure 7.1.  A Civil Defense helmet from the Cold War era. This is not your father's Civil Defense!

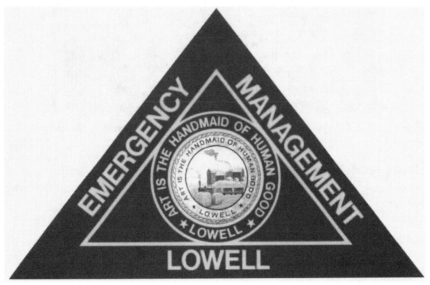

Figure 7.2.  A New EM logo (Lowell, MA) indicates the new Emergency Management vs. Civil Defense.

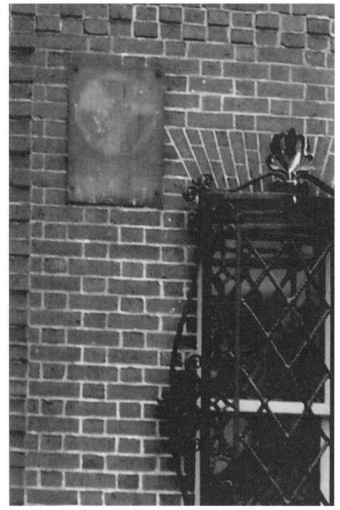

**Figure 7.3.   A faded fallout shelter sign on a building. Pets were not allowed here.**

When any storm is named, everyone in the potential path of the storm should take it seriously. They should watch it closely and begin the implementation of their family disaster plan.

### Why Pet Owners Must Plan

Some public hurricane refuges still will not accept pets. If citizens wait until the last minute to evacuate, they may have no choice but to go to a public refuge that

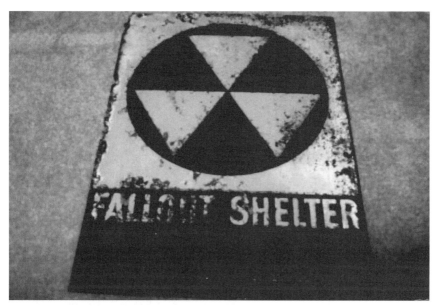

**Figure 7.4.  A close-up shot of a fallout shelter sign.**

doesn't accept pets. If such a situation forces your citizens to leave pets behind, emergency managers can help by advising them to prepare their children and other family members for the fact that the pets may not survive or may be irretrievably lost before people are able or permitted to return to their homes. It's not a pleasant thought but one that managers can help prepare people for.

There is no way to know how long it will be before people are permitted back after the storm. Frightened animals can quickly slip out open doors, broken windows, or other areas of a home that has suffered damage by a vicious storm. Released pets are likely to die of exposure, starvation, predators, or contaminated food or water; on the road, they can run into problems themselves or endanger others. In shelters that do accept pets, even normally friendly animals of different species should not be allowed together unattended, since the stress of the storm may cause distinct behavior changes.

If people are evacuating, conditions are not only unsafe for them but unsafe for other living creatures as well!

### Develop a Written Plan

A written plan will help pet owners and their pets survive. Emergency managers can advise pet owners to identify their evacuation zone and elevation to determine whether they would have to evacuate, and when. If pet owners are located on the storm surge flood plain, the decision to evacuate will always depend on the category and severity of the storm. A good rule of thumb is to always prepare for one category stronger than what is being forecast, as, many times, hurricanes strengthen just before making landfall.

What people do with pets depends on where they and their family will be going in the event of a storm or hurricane. Joining friends and family in a safe location is the preferred option. People should talk over where and how pets will be housed. If they plan to stay in a motel or hotel, they should call ahead of time to determine any restrictions. Some motels and hotels require deposits.

When people are planning to board their pets, a good tip is to survey the kennels to determine specific locations and requirements. Most boarding facilities require proof of up-to-date vaccinations and also require reservations, especially during storms. Remember that some public shelters do not allow pets because they have no place to care for them. Many communities are now dealing with this issue and are trying to allow pet owners the ability to have their pets remain with them. This will take some time to change, so in the meantime, pet owners should be encouraged to evacuate early and go to a shelter where pets are accepted. Pet owners can check with the animal services department for options available in their area. Most areas have some type of plan that will include pets.

The pet owner's goal should be to evacuate to a safe location as close as reasonable to his or her home. If it can be avoided safely, long-distance evacuation is not recommended because highways can be crowded. Friends or relatives in a safe area are the best choice. (Get the word out in newsletters and cable TV to advise people of this well in advance of a storm.) For pet owners, the comfort of knowing they are safe together far outweighs any inconvenience. If a shelter is necessary and it is unable to house both owner and pets, the owner can try to arrange shelter for pets at a veterinary office or kennel close to their evacuation location so the owner will be able to have as much contact with them as possible. Owners and their pets will fare better if they are together.

All animals should have secure carriers (or collapsible cages for large dogs), as well as collars, leashes, and current rabies tags. Carriers should be large enough for the animals to stand comfortably and turn around.

Before the hurricane season begins on June 1 of each year, make sure to get the word out to pet owners to ensure that all of their pets have current immunizations and advise the owners to take these records with them if they must evacuate. It's a good idea to remind pet owners to photograph each of their pets prior to storm season and include these pictures with immunization and allergy records.

Emergency managers that have shelters that accept pets should encourage pet owners to have a pet survival kit. The pet survival kit should include ample food (at least a two-week supply); water/food bowls; medications; specific care instructions; newspapers and plastic trash bags for handling waste; brushes,

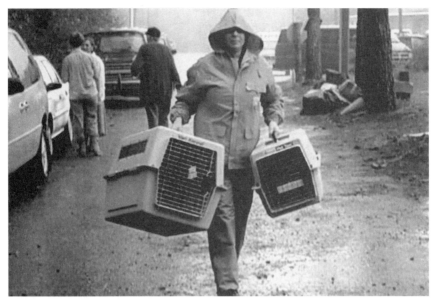

**Figure 7.5.** It's always better to have owners and pets together. Don't forget the cages/carriers.

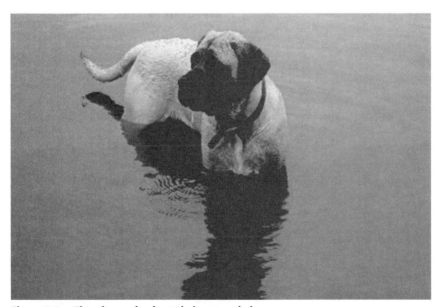

**Figure 7.6.** The aftermath of pets being stranded.

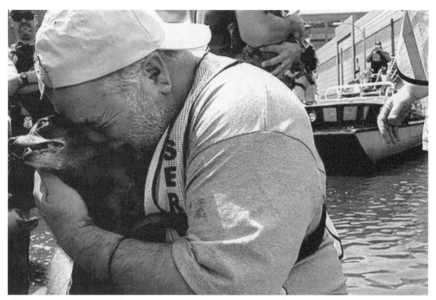

**Figure 7.7.   An emergency worker rescues a pet and shares an emotional moment.**

combs, and other hygiene items; toys and other comfort items; and muzzles if necessary. A manual can opener is a necessity. All belongings should be clearly marked with identification.

Your staff should take first-aid and CPR courses and keep the manuals handy. The same basic principles apply to animals. Ask an area veterinarian for an emergency care pamphlet for animals.

If people have exotic pets, they might want to contact local pet stores or zoological societies, in a safe area, for assistance in sheltering pets. Again, owners should be prepared to supply appropriate housing (not glass) and other necessary supplies to sustain the pet for at least two weeks.

The pet shelter facility should be operated by knowledgeable and capable staff, and the location should be high and dry and of sturdy construction.

## Planning for the Future

Emergency management and health officials across the nation are preparing plans to include pets in disaster planning. According to the District of Columbia Department of Health, working with the D.C. Emergency Management Agency and The Humane Society of the United States, they were one of the first agencies in the country to sign official documents (see www.dc.gov). The signing comes two months after President Bush signed legislation that requires states and local governments to draw up plans to include pets in disaster planning.

A poll conducted by Zogby International (www.zogby.com) following Hurricane Katrina found that 61 percent of pet owners said they would not evacuate before a disaster if they could not bring their pets. This is an amazing statistic and one that prompted the president to sign the legislation requiring contingencies for animals.

"After Hurricane Katrina, many residents would not evacuate because they could not take their pets," said Barbara Childs-Pair, director of the D.C. Emergency Management Agency. "This would not happen in the District of Columbia because we have plans in place that allow residents to shelter people with their pets. We also have a very good relationship between government agencies and those humane organizations like The Humane Society of the United States that would assist us with animal protection and care."

Emergency managers must deal closely with the local board of health or other agency that oversees aspects of animal sheltering, including provisions for people with animals. The Humane Society also encourages families with pets to prepare for disaster to strike.

# 8

# International Emergency Management

A S WE HAVE ALREADY MENTIONED, no entity is exempt from a disaster. As we've seen through television, the Internet, and newspapers, disasters occur all around the world, showing the need for emergency management, disaster preparedness, and emergency managers worldwide.

Obviously, in this book we cannot discuss every country, but I want to take a look at a few countries and highlight the efforts they are taking—or perhaps the lack of effort they are making—in the emergency management field.

## Israel's Emergency Management

One need not travel to Israel to see what makes Israel different from many emergency management (EM) programs in the United States. Israel has a constant threat hanging over the country. Many state and local programs in the United States often suffer when the time between the last major disasters reaches five years or so. Many state emergency management agencies and local communities in the United States see interest in their programs start to drop off at that point because elected officials and citizens "forget" about the previous disasters. It seems that sometimes, elected officials are only driven by what's going to happen at the next press conference and they dismiss the fact that a disaster is bound to happen; it's only a matter of time.

With Israel having a disaster quite often (it seems like weekly, at least), the emphasis is on preparedness. Israel does an exceptional job, in my opinion, of getting the message out to the citizens that they need to be prepared. It also seems as if they have officials' support and a sufficient budget to handle the emergencies that frequently occur.

## Scotland's Program

Officials in Scotland have failed to prepare properly for a major disaster such as multiple terrorist attacks or a flu pandemic, according to an article on the Red Orbit website (www.redorbit.com). The report by the Centre for Disaster Management identified "shortcomings in the current plans of the Scottish Executive, emergency services, councils, health and other services."

The report found a number of gaps in emergency planning, including the failure to carry out one mass evacuation exercise. It also accused emergency planners of "misplaced confidence" over emergency measures that are already in place.

Further, the report says that in the event of a local disaster, one of eight Strategic Coordinating Groups (SCG) will coordinate the response. Nationally, in Scotland, the Strategic Emergency Council Committee leads the response.

The report finds that in five of the eight SCGs, emergency plans for a major incident have never been tested but that SCGs were "confident" plans will work. It is hard to believe that emergency managers could be confident in plans that were never tested. The report also sees too much focus among agencies on public order issues in relation to a flu pandemic (not necessarily the *most* important issue in this type of emergency but it is important). There is also a huge concern about a potential shortage of public health and mortuary services. These two services are crucial in a large-scale disaster and without sufficient resources, the disaster can escalate to the next level.

## Australia's Emergency Management

In my opinion, Australia has a decent EM program. The nation's emergency management training needs are identified in consultation with state and territory stakeholders. Expressed training needs are assessed against national competency standards from the public safety and related training packages so that, wherever possible, training is consistent with the national training framework, enabling pathways for career/study progression in the public safety or other industries.

Competency-based curriculum is in the process of being developed to meet training needs that do not align with national competency standards. The curricula will be nationally accredited through the Victorian Qualifications Authority.

Australian EM agencies also offer professional development activities, giving people with emergency management responsibilities the opportunity to keep abreast of the best practices in their field.

They also have an excellent quality assurance programs, and services are continually evaluated and improved to ensure they are responsive to the needs of the government and the citizens.

## Canada's EM Program

On July 16–18, 2000, the Eastern Canadian Premiers met with the New England Governors in Halifax, Nova Scotia, to sign an agreement entitled International Emergency Management Assistance Memorandum of Understanding. This memorandum was to reinforce an earlier signed agreement, inked in 1998. As you might gather, crossing state boundaries is difficult enough without a mutual-aid agreement. Can you imagine crossing international borders?

## Purpose of Agreement

The agreement was to include any or all of the states of Maine, New Hampshire, Vermont, Massachusetts, Rhode Island, and Connecticut and the Provinces of Québec, New Brunswick, Prince Edward Island, Nova Scotia, and Newfoundland, and such other states and provinces that may have a problem whereby assistance could be given to one or another state or province.

The purpose of this compact was to provide for the possibility of mutual assistance among the jurisdictions entering into the compact in managing any emergency or disaster when the affected jurisdiction or jurisdictions ask for assistance, whether arising from natural disaster, technological hazard, manmade disaster, or civil emergency aspects of resources shortages.

This agreement also provided for the process of planning mechanisms among the agencies responsible and for mutual cooperation, including, if need be, emergency-related exercises, testing, or other training activities using equipment and personnel—with such actions occurring outside actual declared emergency periods. Mutual assistance in this agreement also included the use of emergency forces by mutual agreement among party jurisdictions.

Recently the U.S. Coast Guard and the Canadian counterpart participated in not only oil-spill planning and simulated spill scenarios but an actual response in the northern New England and Canada border.

## Summary

Each and every country needs to plan appropriately for the all-hazards emergency system that the United States is using. This is not to imply that the United States is doing everything perfectly. The United States and its state and local entities also suffer from lack of funding in budgets and not having enough trained people on the ground at times of disasters.

If everyone in the EM field can work toward the core concepts, we'll all be better served and protected.

# 9

# Where Do We Go from Here?
# EM Issues for the Future

A S EMERGENCY MANAGERS, we all know that a major flood, hurricane, tornado, or earthquake affecting our communities is likely over the next several years. Just as likely to occur is a technological disaster. As emergency managers, we certainly need to continue to focus our efforts on preparing for and responding to terrorist events, but let's not forget to budget for other issues and to keep the various hazards in mind. Remember your community's capabilities for dealing with natural hazards. If we in the emergency management community concentrate on the following areas, it is my opinion the communities we represent and protect will be well served.

### Get the Public Involved

Over the years, the general public has played a very limited role in emergency management preparedness. As managers, we need to encourage participation and gain support from the citizens of our communities to get involved in "their" emergency plans and recovery actions. The main focus of public efforts by the early Civil Defense programs and the various Red Cross family programs was to inform and educate the public. However, few people were really involved. With all of the new programs offered by the government agencies and the private sector, we should be promoting the emergency management message. FEMA has the "Are You Ready?" program; the Red Cross has many training opportunities for volunteers. There is Citizens Corps, Volunteers in Police Service (VIPS), Community Emergency Response Team (CERT), Fire Corps, and a host of other programs. When the courses are offered, let the public know by sending a message to

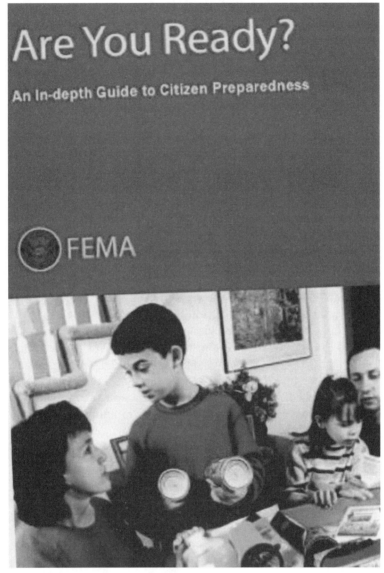

**Figure 9.1.  The FEMA "Are You Ready?" program.**

the local cable access channel or the local newspaper. One community near my town sent out a mailing to every household! That effort was costly but it reaped the results they were looking for. They had so many people sign up for a CERT program, they will be running several this year.

Emergency managers have to engage the public in the emergency preparedness process so that we can fully understand the public's needs and concerns.

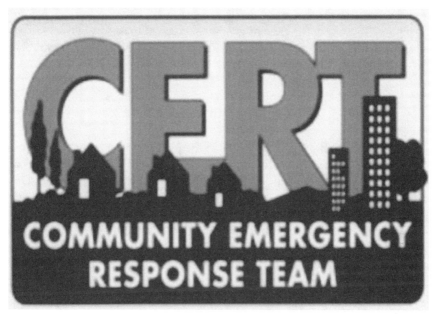

Figure 9.2.   The CERT logo.

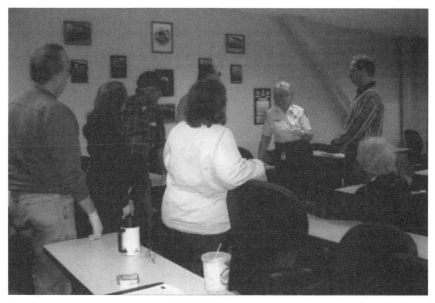

Figure 9.3.   A CERT class prepares the latest group of volunteers for their community.

People have varying concerns during disasters that, perhaps, we do not fully understand. By having the citizens give their input, it makes us better managers and allows us to prepare for disasters and emergencies with a deeper comprehension of the citizens' true needs.

## Remember, It's All Hazards, Now!

While terrorism is always on our minds in the planning process, we must maintain an all-hazards approach to emergency management. Using this approach takes advantage of the general capabilities needed to treat any type of disaster or emergency yet allows for including the special needs of terrorism. If we abandon the all-hazards approach, it would be repeating the mistake the emergency management community made in the 1980s. During the era of the Cold War, FEMA concentrated more than 75 percent of its financial and human resources on preparing for the next nuclear war. FEMA mandated that states and communities receiving federal funding had to spend it according to its formula (75 percent focused on nuclear war capabilities).

As some of us might remember, Hurricanes Hugo, Iniki, and Andrew showed that state and local capabilities were quickly overcome. The federal response under FEMA was somewhat disorganized and a bit late in arriving. In the case of Hurricane Andrew, the director of FEMA was replaced as the in-charge official and the military provided most of the initial support. This true, actual example of the craziness that can result from focusing efforts on just one issue, at the cost of more common and extensive threats, provides strong confirmation of the wisdom of the all-hazards approach to emergency management.

## Try to Establish a Public-Private Partnership

Many people at various levels of the DHS and numerous business groups, such as The Business Roundtable, recognize that a strong partnership between government and business has to be established as part of the country's homeland security efforts. This is important, since almost 85 percent of the infrastructure in this country is privately held!

However, since the September 11 attacks, very few partnerships have been established. There needs to be continued progress and cooperation to incorporate the business sector into the government's emergency management activities—at all levels. The business community must be included in the planning process not only for terrorism but also for natural disasters.

Several large corporations and many small companies have already entered into agreements with governmental agencies to provide assistance in the event of catastrophe. Businesses including Wal-Mart, Target, and Home Depot have already stepped up to the plate and are leading the way in the partnership efforts. Additionally, at DHS, there is a now a computerized list of private resources, called the National Emergency Relief Registry, available to assist emergency managers identify, locate, and contact those companies who have resources available to assist their communities. We already know that we cannot do emergency planning or recovery alone—partner up and spread the word.

### The Key Is Mitigation

Let's face it, without a disaster, it is difficult for emergency managers to show their worth. Mitigation is a constructive role that emergency managers can practice every day, regardless of the size of the community, and not be dependent on an incident to prove their value. Mitigation is practiced by all sectors of a community. In order for mitigation to be effective, it requires emergency managers to develop coalitions within their community. It can often bring together contrasting sides to solve common problems. Mitigation brings the private sector into the emergency management system because economic sustainability of their businesses depends on risk reduction, so mitigation promotes their support and leadership. Mitigation provides the entry point to involve the private sector in other phases of emergency management and to understand their unique needs in the event of a disaster response or recovery operations after an event.

In the late 1990s and early 2000s, *business continuity* and *mitigation planning* were the big buzzwords for emergency management. Economic interest often drives the public's reaction. Mitigation works best at the local level and provides that grassroots effort that can apply political pressure for continued emergency management support.

We need to keep up the efforts to have Congress support the national Flood Insurance Program, the National Earthquake Hazard Reduction Program, and the Hazard Mitigation Grant Program.

### Keep Up with Technology

It isn't easy, with budget cuts and fewer grants available, to keep current with the latest and greatest inventions and technological advances that become available. There are many innovative ideas that become available on a regular basis that emergency managers may be able to take advantage of, including:

- Computer technology (Computer-Aided Management of Emergency Operations—CAMEO; Area Locations of Hazardous Atmospheres—ALOHA)

- Meters and monitors
- Software (inventory, planning, templates, databases)
- Needed equipment

Did you notice that I listed "needed" equipment? I did this for a reason. Often, we hear of a neighboring emergency manager that gets the newest gadget and it was very expensive. We sometimes ask ourselves, "How or why did he buy that thing? What will he use that for?" This is especially true for grant-related items. It is easy to apply for the grants and then, when they are approved, we buy unnecessary items to impress the citizens or show off to the neighboring city or town.

Wouldn't it be great if we were all able to obtain funding for the "super duper whamodyne"? Let's ask ourselves if we really need it and how often will we use it. That should help us weed out the unneeded items and allow us to concentrate on the practical, useful tools.

How many times do we hear of communities that get grant money for their emergency operations center (EOC)? When the grants are being followed up, grant administrators are being taken to task for not properly managing the funds or the equipment. Here are two examples:

- A community needed money for establishing their EOC and spent thousands of dollars on plasma television sets. Unfortunately, none of the televisions made it to the EOC. Instead they were found in the executive offices of department heads of the city.
- Laptop computers are a popular item to be purchased with grant or budget money. After a brief period of time, the computers are not in the office anymore. They do not travel back and forth daily as would be expected. Instead, the managers' families use these computers at home!

These are just a couple of the more common examples of misuse of grant and budget money. While we all realize the importance of staying up-to-date with the latest goodies, use your head and manage resources properly.


### Core Ideas

In my opinion, there are a few core ideas that might help emergency managers in their roles as disaster executives. These ideas are:

1. The spotlight must be on your customers, both internal (department heads and employees of the agencies you represent) and external (citizens of your community).

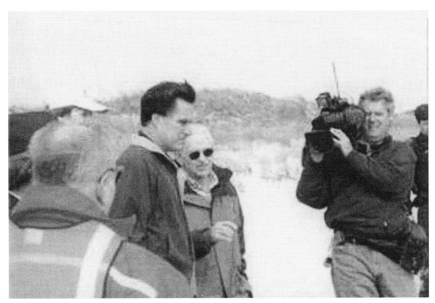

**Figure 9.4. The media covering the former governor of Massachusetts, Mitt Romney, as he is briefed by a state official.**
Courtesy of MADEP.

2. Try to build partnerships among people and agencies, including the private sector and the media. (The media can be your friend or your foe. You make that decision. Remember the press after Hurricane Katrina?)
3. Keep up with and support the development of new technologies to give emergency managers the tools they need to be successful.
4. Keep the public and the media informed.
5. Make mitigation the cornerstone of your program.

These simple, commonsense ideas provide the framework for emergency management to continue to grow and expand its influence, as well as its importance, to the cities and towns and people it serves. Emergency management can ensure its place in the future if the spotlight stays on basic policies, innovative programs, and daily activities that improve the safety and security of individuals and communities.

# Appendix A: Map of FEMA Regions

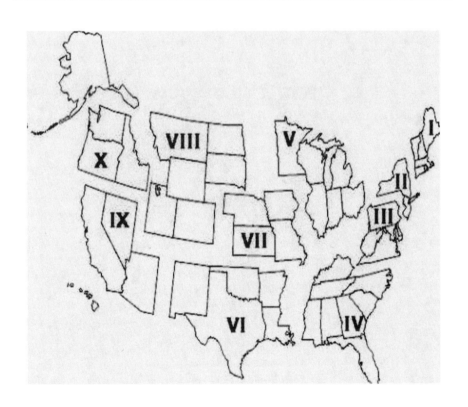

# Appendix B: DHS Organization Chart

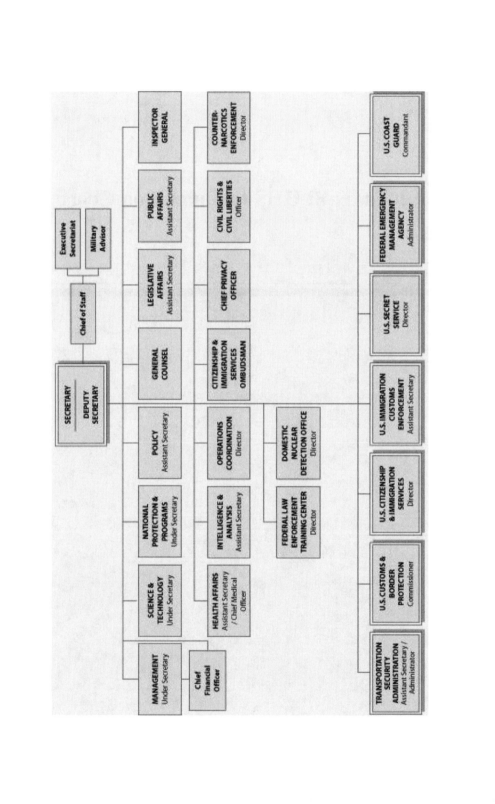

# Appendix C: Emergency Management Logo

The stark insignia of civil defense—a C and D forming a red circle in a white triangle on a blue disk—died yesterday after a long eclipse. It was 67 years old and lived in the mind's eye of anyone who remembers air-raid drills, fallout shelters and metal drums filled with what had to be the stalest biscuits in the world.

Its demise was announced by the National Emergency Management Association, the group that represents state emergency managers. . . .

The [new] EM symbol was endorsed by R. David Paulison, director of the Federal Emergency Management Agency, successor to the civil preparedness agency. He attended the announcement in Washington.

The new image was developed by Morrie Goodman, an emergency communications specialist and the managing director of AGG International, a marketing firm.

"We now have a new symbol of what our profession is all about," Mr. Goodman said.

From "Civil Defense Logo Dies at 67, and Some Mourn Its Passing," David W. Dunlap, *New York Times* December 1, 2006 (http://www.nytimes.com/2006/12/01/washington/01civil.html?_r=3&oref=slogin&oref=slogin&oref=slogin).

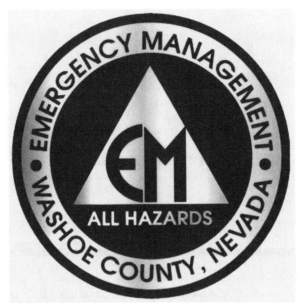

Figure A.3.   A takeoff of the old CD logo, emphasizing the all-hazards approach now part of emergency management.

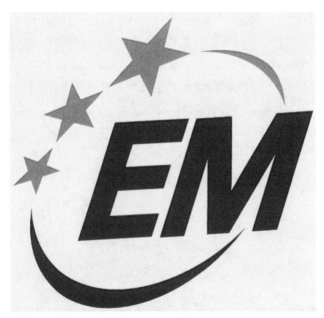

Figure A.4.   The new Emergency Management logo

# Appendix D: Internet Resources

| | |
|---|---|
| All Hands Community | www.all-hands.net |
| Contingency Management Associates, Inc. | www.cmasource.com |
| The Disaster Center | www.disastercenter.com |
| DisasterHelp.gov | www.disasterhelp.gov |
| Disaster Preparedness & Emergency Response Association (DERA) | www.disasters.org/dera/dera.htm |
| Disaster Research Center (Delaware) | www.udel.edu/DRC/index.html |
| Emergency Information Infrastructure Partnership Forum | www.eforum.org |
| International Association of Emergency Planners (IAEM) | www.iaem.com |
| Journal of Homeland Security & Emergency Management | www.bepress.com/jhsem |
| National Emergency Management Association (NEMA) | www.nemaweb.org |
| Precision Planning and Simulations | www.ppscorp.com |
| The International Emergency Management Society (TIEMS) | www.tiems.org |

# Appendix E: Sample City Ordinance Adopting the NIMS

CITY ORDINANCE ADOPTING

THE NATIONAL INCIDENT MANAGEMENT SYSTEM (NIMS)

ORDINANCE NO. _____

AN ORDINANCE ADOPTING THE NATIONAL INCIDENT MANAGEMENT SYSTEM (NIMS) AS THE STANDARD FOR INCIDENT MANAGEMENT BY THE CITY OF _____.

WHEREAS, on February 28, 2003, the President issued Homeland Security Presidential Directive (HSPD)—5 that directed the Department of Homeland Security, in cooperation with representatives of federal, state, and local government, to develop a National Incident Management System (NIMS) to provide a consistent approach to the effective management of situations involving natural disasters, man-made disasters or terrorism; and

WHEREAS, the final NIMS was released on March 1, 2004, and

WHEREAS, the NIMS contains a practice model for the accomplishment of the significant responsibilities associated with prevention, preparedness, response, recovery, and mitigation of all major and national hazards situations, and

WHEREAS, the HSPD-5 requires that state and local governments adopt the NIMS by fiscal year 2005 as a pre-condition to the receipt of federal grants, contract and activities related to the management and preparedness for certain disaster and hazard situations; and

WHEREAS, the City Council for the City of _____ desires to adopt the NIMS as required by HSPD-5.

NOW, THEREFORE, BE IT RESOLVED BY THE CITY COUNCIL OF THE CITY OF _____:

Hereby adopts the National Incident Management System dated March 1, 2004.

READ AND APPROVED on first reading this the ___ day of _____, 20_____.

READ AND APPROVED AND ADOPTED on second reading this the ___ day of _____, 20_____.

_____

, Mayor

City of _____, State

ATTEST:

_____

, Secretary

# Appendix F: Emergency Support Functions under the National Response Plan

| ESF | | | SCOPE |
|---|---|---|---|
| #1—Transportation | | | • Federal and civil transportation support |
| | Coordinator: | DOT | • Transportation Safety |
| | Primary Agency: | DOT | • Restoration/recovery of transportation |
| | Support Agencies: | BTS, DOD, DOS, GSA, IAIP, USCG, USPS | infrastructure |
| #2—Communications | | | • Coordinate with Telecommunication Industry |
| | Coordinator: | DHS/NCS | • Restoration/repair of telecommunication network |
| | Primary Agency: | DHS/NCS | • Cyber and Information Technology |
| | Support Agencies: | DOC, DOD, DOI, FCC, FEMA, GSA, IAIP, S&T, USFS | |
| #3—Public Works and Engineering | | | • Infrastructure protection and emergency repair |
| | Coordinator: | DOD/USACE | • Infrastructure restoration |
| | Primary Agencies: | USACE / FEMA / IAIP | • Engineering services, Construction Management |
| | Support Agencies: | DOC, DOD, DOI, DOL, DOT, EPA, HHS, TVA, USDA, VA | • Critical Infrastructure Liaison |
| #4—Firefighting | | | • Firefighting activities on federal lands |
| | Coordinator: | USFS/USDA | • Resource support to rural and urban firefight operations |
| | Primary Agency: | USFS/USDA | |
| | Support Agencies: | DOD, DOI, EPA, USFA | |
| #5—Emergency Management | | | • Information collection, analysis and reports |
| | Coordinator: | DHS/EPR/FEMA | • Action planning and tracking |
| | Primary Agency: | DHS/EPR/FEMA | • Resource tracking |
| | Support Agencies: | ARC, BTS, DOC, DOD, DOEd, DOE, DOI, DOT, EPA, GSA, HHS, NCS, NASA, NRC, TREAS, SBA, USCG, USDA | • Science and Technology support |

#6—Mass Care, Housing & Human Services
    Coordinator: DHS/EPR/FEMA
    Primary Agencies: DHS/EPR/FEMA /ARC
    Support Agencies: DHS, DOD, DOE, GSA, HHS, HUD, SBA, USDA, USPS, VA

- Mass Care
- Disaster Housing
- Human Services

#7—Resource Support
    Coordinator: GSA
    Primary Agency: GSA/FEMA
    Support Agencies: BTS, DOC, DOD, DOE, DOL, DOT, NASA, OPM, VA, USFS

- Resource Support
- Logistics

#8—Public Health and Medical Services
    Coordinator: HHS
    Primary Agency: HHS
    Support Agencies: FEMA, AID, DHS, DOD, DOE, DOJ, DOL, DOS, DOT, EPA, GSA, USDA, USPS, VA

- Public Health
- Medical
- Mass Fatalities

#9—Urban Search and Rescue
    Coordinator: DHS/EPR/FEMA
    Primary Agency: DHS/EPR/FEMA
    Support Agencies: AID, BTS, DOC, DOD, DOJ, DOL, HHS, NASA, USFS, USCG

- Life saving assistance
- Urban search and rescue

#10—Oil and Hazardous Materials Response
    Coordinator: EPA
    Primary Agencies: EPA (Inland) / USCG (Coastal)
    Support Agencies: DOD, DOE, DOI, DOJ, DOS, DOT, FEMA, GSA, HHS, IAIP, NOAA, NRC, OSHA, S&T, TREAS, USDA

- Hazardous materials (hazardous substances, oil, and the like) response
- Environmental safety and cleanup

(continues)

| ESF | | | SCOPE |
|---|---|---|---|
| #11—Agriculture and Natural Resources | | | • Nutritional services |
| | Coordinator: | DOI/USDA | • Agricultural production |
| | Primary Agency: | DOI/USDA | • Animal health |
| | Support Agencies: | ARC, DOD, DOS, EPA, GSA, IAIP, S&T | |
| #12—Energy | | | • Energy system assessment |
| | Coordinator: | DOE | • Repair/restoration |
| | Primary Agency: | DOE | • Energy industry utilities coordination |
| | Support Agencies: | DHS, DOD, DOI, DOS, DOT, NRC, TVA, USDA, IAIP | • Energy forecast |
| #13—Public Safety and Security | | | • Operational and personnel security |
| | Coordinator: | DOI/DHS/EPR/FEMA | • Liaison between criminal investigation activities and response and recovery operations |
| | Primary Agency: | DOI/DHS/EPR/FEMA | |
| | Support Agencies: | BTS, DOE, DOI, IAIP, USCG, USDA, USPS, USSS | • Inspector General activities |
| #14—Long Term Community Recovery and Mitigation | | | • Assess economic impacts |
| | Coordinator: | FEMA/DHS/EPR | • Private sector coordination |
| | Primary Agencies: | FEMA/DOC/HUD/TREAS/SBA/HHS/DHS/DOD, | • Long-term community recovery |
| | Support Agencies: | DOL, DHS, HHS, IAIP, TVA, USDA, Private Sector | • Mitigation response and program implementation |
| #15—External Affairs | | | * Emergency public information |
| | Coordinator: | DHS | • Protective action guidance |
| | Primary Agency: | FEMA/DHS/EPR | • Media Relations |
| | Support Agencies: | DOC, DOD, DOE, DOI, DOJ, DOL, DOT, DOS, EPA, GSA, HHS, NRC, USDA | • Community Relations |
| | | | • Congressional Affairs |
| | | | • International Affairs |

## Emergency Support Functions (ESF)

- ESF 1—Transportation
  - Responsible for coordinating transportation support to governments and voluntary organizations. Transportation support includes the following:
    - (1) performance of and assisting with evacuation and reentry;
    - (2) processing of all transportation assistance requests and tasks received in the EOC;
    - (3) prioritizing transportation resources for the transportation of people, materials, and services;
    - (4) performing all necessary actions to assist with recovery operations.
  - Federal Lead Agency: U.S. Department of Transportation

- ESF 2—Communications
  - Responsible for coordinating actions to be taken to assure the provision of required communications (two-way radios) and telecommunications (computer and telephone systems) support to disaster personnel. Activation of warning systems and restoration of essential communication systems are coordinated by ESF 2.
  - Federal Lead Agency: U.S. National Communications System

- ESF 3—Public Works
  - Responsible for providing technical advice and evaluations, engineering systems, construction management and inspection, emergency contacting, emergency repair of wastewater and solid waste facilities, removal and handling of debris, and the opening and maintaining of roadways.
  - Federal Lead Agency: U.S. Department of Defense, U.S. Army Corps of Engineers

- ESF 4—Firefighting
  - Responsible for firefighting activities and support services including training, suppression, investigations, and code compliance. Areas of responsibility and activities include suburban, urban, rural, and wildland settings and the interface between each environment.
  - Federal Lead Agency: U.S. Department of Agriculture, Forest Service

- ESF 5—Information and Planning
  - Responsible for collecting, processing, and disseminating information to facilitate emergency response and recovery efforts. Preparation of special operations plans and damage and needs assessments are handled by ESF 5.
  - Federal Lead Agency: Federal Emergency Management Agency

- ESF 6—Mass Care
  - Responsible for coordinating efforts to provide shelter, food, and emergency first aid and for coordinating bulk distribution of emergency relief supplies to disaster victims.
  - Federal Lead Agency: American Red Cross

- ESF 7—Resource Support
  - Responsible for providing logistical and resource support to entities involved in delivering emergency response efforts for natural and technological disasters.
  - Federal Lead Agency: U.S. General Services Administration

- ESF 8—Health and Medical
  - Responsible for coordinating health and medical resources needed to respond to public health and medical care needs prior to, during, and following a disaster.
  - Federal Lead Agency: U.S. Department of Health and Human Services

- ESF 9—Search and Rescue
  - Responsibilities include searching for and locating disaster victims in urban, suburban, and rural environments.
  - Federal Lead Agency: Federal Emergency Management Agency

- ESF 10—Hazardous Materials
  - Responsibilities include coordination in response to an actual or potential discharge and/or release of hazardous materials resulting from a natural or technological disasters.
  - Federal Lead Agency: U.S. Environmental Protection Agency

- ESF 11—Food and Water
  - Responsibilities include identifying, securing, and arranging for coordinating the transport of food and water assistance to affected areas.
  - Federal Lead Agency: U.S. Department of Agriculture, Food and Nutrition Services

- ESF 12—Energy
  - Responsible for coordinating the provision of emergency power to support emergency response and recovery efforts and normalized community functions. ESF 12 provides electric power, distribution systems, fuel, and emergency generators.
  - Federal Lead Agency: U.S. Department of Energy

- ESF 13—Military Support
  - Responsibilities include outlining specific tasks, resources, locations, and responsibilities to support the military presence in county during disaster operations.

- ESF 14—Public Information
  - Responsible for coordinating emergency public warning and information systems.

- ESF 15—Volunteers and Donations
  - Responsibilities include expediting the delivery of voluntary goods and services supporting relief efforts before and after a disaster impact.

- ESF 16—Law Enforcement
  - Responsibilities include establishing procedures for the command, control, and coordination of law enforcement agencies to support disaster response operations. ESF 16 works with the National Guard in support of security missions and other law enforcement agency activities.

- ESF 17—Animal Services
  - Responsible for coordinating all animal response and relief activities.

# Appendix G: Volunteer Application

Personal Information:

Name: _____

Address: _____

Phone Numbers: _____

E-mail Address: _____

Employment Information (Title, Place of Employment): _____
_____

Emergency Contact Information (Name, Phone Numbers): _____
_____

Describe any restrictions on your activities (physical, medical, mental): _____
_____

Date of last tetanus shot: _____

General Availability:

| | Sunday | Monday | Tuesday | Wednesday | Thursday | Friday | Saturday |
|---|---|---|---|---|---|---|---|
| AM | | | | | | | |
| PM | | | | | | | |

Do you have personal transportation: _____

Are you willing/able to do manual labor:     ☐ Yes      ☐ No

Skills & Qualifications:

Fluency in Language(s) other than English: _____

Licenses/Professional Certification: _____
_____

Professional Background: _____
_____

Education Background: _____
_____

Computer Skills: _____
_____

Prior or Current Volunteer Experience: _____
_____

Prior Disaster Relief Experience: _____
_____

Other Skills:

☐ Administrative/Secretarial
☐ Accounting/Finance/Bookkeeping
☐ Civil Servant
☐ Child Care
☐ Customer Service
☐ Food Service
☐ Health Services (Doctor, Nurse, EMT)
☐ Transportation (Professional Truck/ Bus Driver)

☐ Human Resources (interviewing, recruiting)
☐ Mental Health Counselor/ Social Worker
☐ Management
☐ Technical
☐ Trade:_____
☐ Other:_____

Volunteer Agreement:
1. The information provided is complete and true. If information given on this application is incomplete or untrue, I understand my assignment may be terminated.
2. I understand that my own insurance will be used as coverage for illnesses and injuries and that I am ultimately responsible for any costs incurred in my volunteer efforts.
3. I agree to respect the rights, property, and confidentiality of emergency workers, agencies involved and individuals affected by disaster.
4. I agree to adhere to the rules/instructions of my job assignment(s) so as not to jeopardize emergency operations or procedures.

Signature: _____

Date: _____

# Appendix H: Emergency Management Agency Volunteer Application

| PERSONAL INFORMATION | | |
|---|---|---|
| Last Name | First Name (middle initial) | |
| Address | | |
| City | State | Zip Code |
| Date of Birth | Drivers License Number | |
| Home Phone | Cell Phone | |
| EMPLOYMENT INFORMATION | | |
| Current Employer | Supervisor | |
| Address | | |
| City | State | Zip Code |
| Work Phone | | |
| Work Responsibilities | | |
| Immediate Past Employer | Supervisor | |
| Work Responsibilities | | |
| Past Employer | Supervisor | |
| Work Responsibilities | | |

| AGENCY INTEREST | |
|---|---|
| Division Applying For | |

| PROFESSIONAL LICENSES | |
|---|---|
| License | Number and State of Issue |
| License | Number and State of Issue |
| License | Number and State of Issue |

| SKILLS & QUALIFICATIONS & APPLICABLE TRAINING |
|---|
| |
| |
| |

| REFERENCES | |
|---|---|
| Name | Years Known |
| Phone Number | Relationship |
| Name | Years Known |
| Phone Number | Relationship |
| Name | Years Known |
| Phone Number | Relationship |

| LEGAL |
|---|
| Have you even been convicted of any felony or misdemeanor other than minor traffic violations? |
| If yes, provide details |

## Applicant Statement

I certify that the information I have provided in this application is true and complete to the best of my knowledge. I understand that if my answers are found to be untruthful, my application may be rejected, or if I am already a member of the Emergency Management Agency, any falsifications or misrepresentations on this application may be grounds for dismissal from the membership. I also certify that I am 18 years of age or older, and am a legal United States citizen.

I understand that the Emergency Management Agency performs criminal background checks, personal reference checks, and driving record checks on applicants prior to acceptance of membership, and I release the information contained in this application authorizing the Emergency Management Agency to proceed with and receive information from the background check, and that all such information collected during the check will be kept confidential.

I further understand that I do not have to agree to these background checks, but refusal to do so may exclude me from consideration for some types of volunteer positions.

_____

Signature of Applicant

_____

Date

# Appendix I: Emergency Supply Kit

Emergency managers are often asked about preparing emergency supply kits. This listing can help your citizens in setting up their kits. When preparing for emergency situations, it's best to have folks think first about the basics of their survival.

### Basic Necessities

- Fresh water
- Food
- Clean air
- Warmth

### Recommended Supply List

- Battery-operated AM/FM radio and extra batteries
- Sunscreen
- ChapStick with sunscreen
- Poncho
- Toilet paper
- Ziploc bags
- Twelve-hour light sticks
- Flashlight
- Insect repellent
- Space blankets

- Survival food: High-calorie food bars or Meals Ready to Eat (MREs)
- First-aid kit
- Spark-free wrench for shutting off natural gas
- Safety goggles
- Filter masks or dust masks
- Playing cards (to kill boredom, draw lots, mark areas)
- Duct tape
- Heavy leather work gloves
- Hand sanitizer
- Water (one gallon per person per day)
- Nonperishable, ready-to-eat canned foods, and a manual can opener
- Paper cups and plates and plastic utensils
- Whistle (to signal for help)
- Dust or filter masks
- Basic tools (wrench, pliers, screwdrivers, hammer)
- Plastic sheeting
- Garbage bags and plastic ties for personal sanitation
- Extra set of car, building, and business keys
- Personal hygiene items: soap, feminine products, toothbrush, toothpaste, moist towelettes, and the like

### Business Go Bag

Every business should assemble a Business Go Bag—a collection of items you and your employees may need in the event of an evacuation. Encourage employees to have their own portable kits customized to meet personal needs.

**Recommended items include:**
- Battery-operated AM/FM radio and extra batteries
- Flashlight
- Bottled water and nonperishable food such as energy or granola bars
- First-aid kit
- Lightweight raingear and Mylar blankets
- Contact information for emergency personnel
- A small regional map

# Appendix J: Severe Weather Manager's Checklist

- ☐ Reviewed policy, and developed/revised Departmental Preparedness Plan and staffing contingency plan.
- ☐ Reviewed and assigned severe weather/emergency conditions job/work category assignments to staff members.
  - **Essential Service:** In Severe Weather/Emergency Conditions/State of Emergency,
    - ○ report to or remain at work;
    - ○ transportation services provided as necessary; and
    - ○ childcare services provided as available.

  - **Reserve Service:** In Severe Weather/Emergency Conditions/State of Emergency,
    - ○ category assigned at time of each event.

  - **Delayed Service:** In Severe Weather/Emergency Conditions/State of Emergency,
    - ○ do not report to or remain at work;
    - ○ no transportation services provided; and
    - ○ no childcare services provided.
- ☐ Provided an updated list of department staff members' telephone numbers, pagers, and cellular telephone numbers to all staff members.

☐ Reviewed where to obtain information about weather-related/emergency conditions information, including website and telephone numbers.
- _____ **Medical Center / Hospital**
  - ○ _____
- **www.** _____

## Essential Service Category Only

☐ Reviewed specific needs of all categories with my supervisor. Staff members assigned to the Essential Service category may need to plan to potentially spend several days on-site. Preparation kit needs include:

| | |
|---|---|
| Appropriate clothing for three days | Battery alarm clock |
| Toiletries | Back up glasses |
| Flashlight | Cell phone and charger |
| Prescribed medications | Small radio |

# Appendix K: Emergency Manager Checklist: Emergency Response Plan

| Requirements | Completed | Team Member(s) Assigned | Comments |
|---|---|---|---|
| 1. Has an Emergency Manager been designated? | | | |
| 2. Is there an Emergency Response Planning Committee? | | | |
| 3. Does the Emergency Response Plan designate supervisors to account for personnel during an emergency? | | | |
| 4. Are there reporting procedures described in the Emergency Response Plan to address all hazards? | | | |
| 5. Does the Emergency Response Plan address alarm systems to notify citizens of emergencies in the community? | | | |
| 6. Does the Emergency Response Plan contain different types of evacuation methods that will be used for various types of emergencies? | | | |
| 7. Is sufficient number of personnel trained to assist the Emergency Manager? | | | |

| | | | | | |
|---|---|---|---|---|---|
| 8. Has a hazard assessment of the community been accomplished?<br><br>ANALYZE CAPABILITIES AND HAZARDS<br>☐ Review agency specific/special plans and procedures<br>☐ Identify critical services and operations<br>☐ Identify internal resources and capabilities<br>☐ Identify external resources<br>☐ List all potential emergencies | | | | | |
| 9. Color coding ID cards to identify ERT member and assignments | | | | | |
| 10. Key boxes: where are they; what keys are in them; who has access to them | | | | | |
| 11. Equipment evaluation for building: evacuation equipment; spill kits for areas that have haz. materials like cleaning supplies and chemicals; fire extinguishers (where are they and who is trained to operate) | | | | | |
| 12. Garage access during emergencies—program access gates? Identify staff to report there to control access? | | | | | |
| 13. Evacuating after hours: identify staff who may be working in areas where the alarm is not heard well | | | | | |

| Requirements | Completed | Team Member(s) Assigned | Comments |
|---|---|---|---|
| During Special Events Evacuation Procedures | | | |
| 14. EOC alarm system: how it works | | | |
| 15. Use of public address/fire panel system: how it works; when to use; who could access; internal and external speakers | | | |
| 16. Use of handheld radios: who should have; what type, available frequency. | | | |
| 17. Written SOPs/procedures to be included in the plan: security responsibilities when alarm activates; other security needs | | | |
| 18. Has an Emergency Response Plan been developed and implemented?<br><br>DEVELOP THE PLAN<br>☐ Include special operations into Plan<br>☐ Emergency response procedures<br>☐ Support documents<br>☐ Establish a training schedule<br>☐ Review, conduct training<br>☐ Obtain final approval<br>☐ Distribute the Plan to all agencies | | | |

| IMPLEMENT THE PLAN<br>☐ Integrate the Plan into other plans<br>☐ Distribute emergency procedures<br>☐ Conduct training and drills<br>☐ Provide training<br>☐ Evaluate and modify the Plan | | | | | | | |
|---|---|---|---|---|---|---|---|
| 19. Does the Emergency Response Plan contain a personnel accountability method? | | | | | | | |
| 20. Are emergency evacuation procedures in place for essential people? | | | | | | | |
| 21. Has the Emergency Manager posted and designated escape routes and assembly points for emergencies? | | | | | | | |
| 22. Staging of personnel during events: front sides and back; relation to Public Safety Command Post | | | | | | | |
| 23. Did all required personnel review the contents of the Plan? | | | | | | | |
| 24. Specific plans for agencies; who should have copies; when updated | | | | | | | |
| 25. Are emergency drills conducted and how often? | | | | | | | |

| Requirements | Completed | Team Member(s) Assigned | Comments |
|---|---|---|---|
| 26. Is the Emergency Response Plan reviewed with all necessary annually? | | | |
| 27. Making plan available electronically on website for community | | | |
| 28. Drill schedule | | | |

# Appendix L: Evacuation/Drill Record and After Action Report

| |
|---|
| 1. Address/Location of Drill: |
| 2. Date of Drill:                        3. Time of Drill: |
| 4. Time it Took to Evacuate Building: |
| 5. Number of Monitors Available: |
| 6. Specific Problems Encountered: |
| 7. Weather Conditions at the Time of Evacuation/Drill: |
| 8. Estimate Number of Employees Evacuated: |
| 9. Estimate Number of Citizens Evacuated: |
| 10. Specific Tasks Completed: |
| 11. Summary/Recommendations: |
| 12. Emergency Response Coordinator: |

# Appendix M: State Offices and Agencies of Emergency Management

## Federal

**FEMA**
500 C Street SW
Washington, DC 20472
Disaster Assistance: (800) 621-FEMA,
  TTY (800) 462-7585

## A

**Alabama Emergency
  Management Agency**
5898 County Road 41
P.O. Drawer 2160
Clanton, AL 35046-2160
(205) 280-2200
(205) 280-2495 FAX
ema.alabama.gov/

**Alaska Division of
  Emergency Services**
P.O. Box 5750
Fort Richardson, AK 99505-5750

(907) 428-7000
(907) 428-7009 FAX
www.ak-prepared.com

**American Samoa Territorial
  Emergency Management
  Coordination (TEMCO)**
American Samoa Government
P.O. Box 1086
Pago Pago, American Samoa 96799
(011)(684) 699-6415
(011)(684) 699-6414 FAX

**Arizona Division of
  Emergency Management**
5636 E. McDowell Rd
Phoenix, AZ 85008
(602) 244-0504 or 1-800-411-2336
www.azdema.gov

**Arkansas Department of
  Emergency Management**
P.O. Box 758
Conway, AR 72033

(501) 730-9750
(501) 730-9754 FAX
www.adem.state.ar.us/


## C

**California Governor's Office
of Emergency Services**
3650 Schriever Ave.
Mather, CA 95655-4203
(916) 845-8510
(916) 845-8511 FAX
www.oes.ca.gov/

**Colorado Office of
Emergency Management**
Division of Local Government
Department of Local Affairs
9195 East Mineral Avenue
Suite 200
Centennial, CO 80112
(720) 852-6600
(720) 852-6750 Fax
www.dola.state.co.us/oem/
oemindex.htm

**Connecticut Office of
Emergency Management**
Military Department
360 Broad Street
Hartford, CT 06105
(860) 566-3180
(860) 247-0664 FAX
www.mil.state.ct.us/OEM.htm


## D

**Delaware Emergency
Management Agency**
165 Brick Store Landing Road
Smyrna, DE 19977

(302) 659-3362
(302) 659-6855 FAX
www.state.de.us/dema/index.htm

**District of Columbia Emergency
Management Agency**
2000 14th Street, NW, 8th Floor
Washington, DC 20009
(202) 727-6161
(202) 673-2290 FAX
dcema.dc.gov


## F

**Florida Division of
Emergency Management**
2555 Shumard Oak Blvd.
Tallahassee, FL 32399-2100
(850) 413-9969
(850) 488-1016 FAX
floridadisaster.org


## G

**Georgia Emergency
Management Agency**
P.O. Box 18055
Atlanta, GA 30316-0055
(404) 635-7000
(404) 635-7205 FAX
www.State.Ga.US/GEMA/

**Office of Civil Defense**
Government of Guam
P.O. Box 2877
Hagatna, Guam 96932
(011)(671) 475-9600
(011)(671) 477-3727 FAX
http://ns.gov.gu/

**Guam Homeland Security/Office of
Civil Defense**
221B Chalan Palasyo
Agana Heights, Guam 96910

(671) 475-9600
(671) 477-3727
www.guamhs.org

## H

**Hawaii State Civil Defense**
3949 Diamond Head Road
Honolulu, HI 96816-4495
(808) 733-4300
(808) 733-4287 FAX
www.scd.hawaii.gov

## I

**Idaho Bureau of Disaster Services**
4040 Guard Street, Bldg. 600
Boise, ID 83705-5004
(208) 334-3460
(208) 334-2322 FAX
www2.state.id.us/bds/

**Illinois Emergency**
 **Management Agency**
110 East Adams Street
Springfield, IL 62701
(217) 782-2700
(217) 524-7967 FAX
www.state.il.us/iema

**Indiana State Emergency**
 **Management Agency**
302 West Washington Street
Room E-208 A
Indianapolis, IN 46204-2767
(317) 232-3986
(317) 232-3895 FAX
www.ai.org/sema/index.html

**Iowa Homeland Security &**
 **Emergency Management Division**
Department of Public Defense

Hoover Office Building
Des Moines, IA 50319
(515) 281-3231
(515) 281-7539 FAX
Iowahomelandsecurity.org

## K

**Kansas Division of**
 **Emergency Management**
2800 S.W. Topeka Boulevard
Topeka, KS 66611-1287
(785) 274-1401
(785) 274-1426 FAX
www.ink.org/public/kdem/

**Kentucky Emergency Management**
EOC Building
100 Minuteman Parkway Bldg. 100
Frankfort, KY 40601-6168
(502) 607-1682
(502) 607-1614 FAX
kyem.ky.gov/

## L

**Louisiana Office of**
 **Emergency Preparedness**
7667 Independence Blvd.
Baton Rouge, LA 70806
(225) 925-7500
(225) 925-7501 FAX
www.ohsep.louisiana.gov

## M

**Maine Emergency**
 **Management Agency**
45 Commerce Drive, Suite #2
#72 State House Station
Augusta, ME 04333-0072
(207) 624-4400

(207) 287-3180 (FAX)
www.state.me.us/mema/
  memahome.htm

**CNMI Emergency**
  **Management Office**
Office of the Governor
Commonwealth of the Northern
  Mariana Islands
P.O. Box 10007
Saipan, Mariana Islands 96950
(670) 322-9529
(670) 322-7743 FAX
www.cnmiemo.org/

**National Disaster**
  **Management Office**
Office of the Chief Secretary
P.O. Box 15
Majuro, Republic of the Marshall
  Islands 96960-0015
(011)(692) 625-5181
(011)(692) 625-6896 FAX

**Maryland Emergency**
  **Management Agency**
Camp Fretterd Military Reservation
5401 Rue Saint Lo Drive
Reistertown, MD 21136
(410) 517-3600
(877) 636-2872 Toll-Free
(410) 517-3610 FAX
www.mema.state.md.us/

**Massachusetts Emergency**
  **Management Agency**
400 Worcester Road
Framingham, MA 01702-5399
(508) 820-2000
(508) 820-2030 FAX
www.state.ma.us/mema

**Michigan Division of**
  **Emergency Management**
4000 Collins Road
P.O. Box 30636
Lansing, MI 48909-8136
(517) 333-5042
(517) 333-4987 FAX
www.michigan.gov/msp/
  1,1607,7-123-1593_3507---,00.html

**National Disaster Control Officer**
Federated States of Micronesia
P.O. Box PS-53
Kolonia, Pohnpei
Micronesia 96941
(011)(691) 320-8815
(001)(691) 320-2785 FAX

**Minnesota Homeland Security**
  **and Emergency Management**
Department of Public Safety
Suite 223
444 Cedar Street
St. Paul, MN 55101-6223
(651) 296-2233
(651) 296-0459 FAX
www.hsem.state.mn.us/

**Mississippi Emergency**
  **Management Agency**
P.O. Box 4501—Fondren Station
Jackson, MS 39296-4501
(601) 352-9100
(800) 442-6362 Toll Free
(601) 352-8314 FAX
www.www.msema.org
www.msema.org/mitigate/
  mssaferoominit.htm

**Missouri Emergency**
  **Management Agency**
P.O. Box 116

2302 Militia Drive
Jefferson City, MO 65102
(573) 526-9100
(573) 634-7966 FAX
sema.dps.mo.gov

**Montana Division of Disaster &**
**Emergency Services**
1900 Williams Street
Helena, MT 59604-4789
(406) 841-3911
(406) 444-3965 FAX
dma.mt.gov/des/


**N**

**Nebraska Emergency**
**Management Agency**
1300 Military Road
Lincoln, NE 68508-1090
(402) 471-7410
(402) 471-7433 FAX
www.nema.ne.gov

**Nevada Division of**
**Emergency Management**
2525 South Carson Street
Carson City, NV 89711
(775) 687-4240
(775) 687-6788 FAX
dem.state.nv.us/

**Governor's Office of**
**Emergency Management**
State Office Park South
107 Pleasant Street
Concord, NH 03301
(603) 271-2231
(603) 225-7341 FAX
www.nhoem.state.nh.us/

**New Jersey Office of**
**Emergency Management**
Emergency Management Bureau
P.O. Box 7068
West Trenton, NJ 08628-0068
(609) 538-6050 Monday-Friday
(609) 882-2000 ext 6311 (24/7)
(609) 538-0345 FAX
www.state.nj.us/oem/county/

**New Mexico Department**
**of Public Safety**
Office of Emergency Management
P.O. Box 1628
13 Bataan Boulevard
Santa Fe, NM 87505
(505) 476-9600
(505) 476-9635 Emergency
(505) 476-9695 FAX
www.dps.nm.org/emergency/
index.htm

**Emergency Management Bureau**
Department of Public Safety
P.O. Box 1628
13 Bataan Boulevard
Santa Fe, NM 87505
(505) 476-9606
(505) 476-9650
www.dps.nm.org/emc.htm

**New York State Emergency**
**Management Office**
1220 Washington Avenue
Building 22, Suite 101
Albany, NY 12226-2251
(518) 457-2222
(518) 457-9995 FAX
www.nysemo.state.ny.us/

**North Carolina Division of**
**Emergency Management**
4713 Mail Service Center

Raleigh, NC 27699-4713
(919) 733-3867
(919) 733-5406 FAX
www.dem.dcc.state.nc.us/

**North Dakota Division
of Emergency Management**
P.O. Box 5511
Bismarck, ND 58506-5511
(701) 328-8100
(701) 328-8181 FAX
www.state.nd.us/dem


**O**


**Ohio Emergency
Management Agency**
2855 W. Dublin Granville Road
Columbus, OH 43235-2206
(614) 889-7150
(614) 889-7183 FAX
www.state.oh.us/odps/division/ema/

**Office of Civil Emergency
Management**
Will Rogers Sequoia Tunnel
2401 N. Lincoln
Oklahoma City, OK 73152
(405) 521-2481
(405) 521-4053 FAX
www.odcem.state.ok.us/

**Oregon Emergency Management**
Department of State Police
PO Box 14370
Salem, OR 97309-5062
(503) 378-2911
(503) 373-7833 FAX
egov.oregon.gov/OOHS/OEM

**P**

**Palau NEMO Coordinator**
Office of the President
P.O. Box 100
Koror, Republic of Palau 96940
(011)(680) 488-2422
(011)(680) 488-3312

**Pennsylvania Emergency
Management Agency**
2605 Interstate Drive
Harrisburg, PA 17110-9463
(717) 651-2001
(717) 651-2040 FAX
www.pema.state.pa.us/

**Puerto Rico Emergency
Management Agency**
P.O. Box 966597
San Juan, Puerto Rico 00906-6597
(787) 724-0124
(787) 725-4244 FAX


**R**

**Rhode Island Emergency
Management Agency**
645 New London Ave
Cranston, RI 02920-3003
(401) 946-9996
(401) 944-1891 FAX
www.riema.ri.gov


**S**

**South Carolina Emergency
Management Division**
2779 Fish Hatchery Road
West Columbia, SC 29172

(803) 737-8500
(803) 737-8570 FAX
www.scemd.org/

**South Dakota Division
of Emergency Management**
118 West Capitol
Pierre, SD 57501
(605) 773-3231
(605) 773-3580 FAX
www.state.sd.us/dps/sddem/home.htm

### T

**Tennessee Emergency
Management Agency**
3041 Sidco Drive
Nashville, TN 37204-1502
(615) 741-4332
(615) 242-9635 FAX
www.tnema.org

**Texas Division of Emergency
Management**
5805 N. Lamar
Austin, TX 78752
(512) 424-2138
(512) 424-2444 or 7160 FAX
www.txdps.state.tx.us/dem/

### U

**Utah Division of Emergency Services
and Homeland Security**
1110 State Office Building
P.O. Box 141710
Salt Lake City, UT 84114-1710
(801) 538-3400

(801) 538-3770 FAX
www.des.utah.gov

### V

**Vermont Emergency
Management Agency**
Department of Public Safety
Waterbury State Complex
103 South Main Street
Waterbury, VT 05671-2101
(802) 244-8721
(802) 244-8655 FAX
www.dps.state.vt.us/

**Virgin Islands Territorial Emergency
Management—VITEMA**
2-C Contant, A-Q Building
Virgin Islands 00820
(340) 774-2244
(340) 774-1491

**Virginia Department
of Emergency Management**
10501 Trade Court
Richmond, VA 23236-3713
(804) 897-6502
(804) 897-6506
www.vdem.state.va.us

### W

**State of Washington Emergency
Management Division**
Building 20, M/S: TA-20
Camp Murray, WA 98430-5122
(253) 512-7000
(253) 512-7200 FAX
www.emd.wa.gov/

**West Virginia Office of**
**Emergency Services**
Building 1, Room EB-80
1900 Kanawha Boulevard, East
Charleston, WV 25305-0360
(304) 558-5380
(304) 344-4538 FAX
www.wvdhsem.gov

**Wisconsin Emergency Management**
2400 Wright Street
P.O. Box 7865
Madison, WI 53707-7865

(608) 242-3232
(608) 242-3247 FAX
emergencymanagement
 .wi.gov/

**Wyoming Office of**
**Homeland Security**
122 W. 25th Street
Cheyenne, WY 82002
(307) 777-4900
(307) 635-6017 FAX
wyohomelandsecurity.state
 .wy.us

# Appendix N: Common Emergency Management Acronyms

| | |
|---|---|
| ACGIH | American Council of Government Industrial Hygienists |
| ANSI | American National Standards Institute |
| BLEVE | Boiling Liquid Expanding Vapor Explosion |
| BSE | Bovine Spongiform Encephalopathy—"mad cow" disease |
| CA | Cooperative Agreement |
| CAA | Clean Air Act |
| CAO | Chief Administrative Officer |
| CAS | Chemical Abstract Service |
| CBO | Community Based Organization |
| CBR | Chemical, Biological, and Radiological |
| CBRNE | Chemical, Biological, Radiological, Nuclear, and Explosive |
| CDC | Centers for Disease Control and Prevention |
| CERT | Community Emergency Response Team |
| CEM | Comprehensive Emergency Management, also Certified Emergency Manager |
| CERCLA | Comprehensive Environmental Response Compensation and Liability Act |
| CFR | Code of Federal Regulations |
| CIST | Critical Incident Stress Team |
| CSEP | Chemical Stockpile Emergency Preparedness |
| DAT | Damage Assessment Teams |
| DFO | Disaster Field Office |
| DHS | Department of Homeland Security |
| DHHS | Department of Health and Human Services |
| DOT | Department of Transportation |

| | |
|---|---|
| EAL | Emergency Action Level |
| EAP | Emergency Action Plan |
| EHS | Extremely Hazardous Substance |
| EMA | Emergency Management Agency |
| EMF | Emergency Management Functions |
| EMPG | Emergency Management Performance Grants |
| EMS | Emergency Medical Services |
| EOC | Emergency Operations Center |
| EOP | Emergency Operations Plan |
| EPA | U.S. Environmental Protection Agency |
| EPCRA | Emergency Planning and Community Right to Know Act |
| EPZ | Emergency Planning Zone |
| ERP | Emergency Response Plan |
| ERT | Emergency Response Teams |
| ESF | Emergency Support Function |
| FBI | Federal Bureau of Investigation |
| FCO | Federal Coordinating Officer |
| FEC | Facility Emergency Coordinator |
| FECA | Federal Employees Compensation Act |
| FIRM | Flood Insurance Rate Maps |
| FEMA | Federal Emergency Management Agency |
| FY | Fiscal Year |
| GIS | Geographical Information System |
| HAZUS | HAZards US |
| HAZUS–MH | HAZards US–MultiHazard |
| HAZWOPER | Hazardous Waste Operations and Emergency Response |
| HMGP | Hazard Mitigation Grant Program |
| HS Act | Homeland Security Act of 2002 |
| HSPD | Homeland Security Presidential Directive |
| HVA | Hazard/Vulnerability Analysis |
| HVAC | Heating, Ventilation, and Air Conditioning |
| IC | Incident Commander |
| ICS | Incident Command System |
| IDLH | Immediately Dangerous to Life or Health |
| IMS | Incident Management System |
| JIC | Joint Information Center |
| LC-50 | Lethal Concentration to 50 percent of those exposed |
| LD-50 | Lethal Dose to 50 percent of those exposed |
| LEL | Lower Explosive Limit |
| LEMA | Local Emergency Management Agency |
| LEPC | Local Emergency Planning Committee |
| LFL | Lower Flammable Limit |

| | |
|---|---|
| MAA | Mutual-Aid Agreement |
| MAC | Multi-Agency Coordination (system) |
| MMRS | Metropolitan Medical Response System |
| MOA | Memorandum of Agreement |
| MOU | Memorandum of Understanding |
| MSDS | Material Safety Data Sheet |
| NCP | National Contingency Plan |
| NDMS | National Disaster Medical System |
| NEMA | National Emergency Management Association |
| NFIP | National Flood Insurance Program |
| NFPA | National Fire Protection Association |
| NGA | National Governors Association |
| NGO | Non-Governmental Organization |
| NIMS | National Incident Management System |
| NOAA | National Oceanographic and Atmospheric Administration |
| NPO | Non-Profit Organization |
| NRC | Nuclear Regulatory Commission |
| NRP | National Response Plan |
| NWS | National Weather Service |
| OCA | Offsite Consequence Analysis |
| OSHA | Occupational Safety and Health Administration |
| SOP | Standard Operating Procedures |
| PAG | Protective Action Guides |
| PAR | Protective Action Recommendation |
| PTSD | Post-Traumatic Stress Disorder |
| PDD | Presidential Disaster Declaration |
| PIO | Public Information Officer |
| PPA | Performance Partnership Agreement |
| PPE | Personal Protective Equipment |
| REP | Radiological Emergency Planning |
| RIT | Rapid Intervention Team |
| RMP | Risk Management Plan |
| ROP | Recovery Operations Plan |
| SEMA | State Emergency Management Agency |
| SARA | Superfund Amendments and Reauthorization Act |
| SEMS | Standardized Emergency Management System (California) |
| SERC | State Emergency Response Commission |
| SOG | Standard Operating Guideline |
| SOP | Standard Operating Procedure |
| TLV | Threshold Limit Value |
| UASI | Urban Areas Security Initiative |
| UEL | Upper Explosive Limit |

| | |
|---|---|
| UFL | Upper Flammable Limit |
| UN | United Nations |
| UNDRO | United Nations Disaster Relief Organization |
| USAR | Urban Search and Rescue |
| USC | United States Code |
| USGS | U.S. Geological Survey |
| VNAT | Victims' Needs Assessment Team |
| VPA | Volunteer Protection Act of 1997 |
| VZ | Vulnerable Zone |
| WMD | Weapons of Mass Destruction |

# Index

agricultural drought, 52
all-hazards approach: basis of, 20; definition of, 19; FEMA, advantages of, 108
ALOHA. *See* Area Locations of Hazardous Atmospheres
American Nuclear Society (ANS), 70
ANS. *See* American Nuclear Society
Area Locations of Hazardous Atmospheres (ALOHA), 109
"Are You Ready" program, 105, *106*
atomic bomb, 5–6
Australia, emergency management in, 102

The Business Roundtable, 108

CAMEO. *See* Computer-Aided Management of Emergency Operations
Canada, emergency management in, 103
Carter, Jimmy, 11, 68
CD. *See* Civil Defense
CEM. *See* Comprehensive Emergency Management

CERT. *See* Community Emergency Response Team
Chernobyl nuclear power plant, *69*
Childs-Pair, Barbara, 99
Citizen Corps, 105
civil defense (CD): 1950s history of, 6–8; 1960s history of, 8–10; 1970s history of, 10–11; 1980's history of, 11–13; 1990s history of, 13–14; emergency management's evolution from, 14–16; fallout shelter emphasis of, 9; helmet used for, *93*; legislation for, 2–3; logo of, *7*; organizational confusion and, 8; reorganization of, 10–11; USA's history, pre-1950, with, 3–6. *See also* Federal Civil Defense Administration; Office of Civil Defense
CND. *See* Council of National Defense
Coast Guard, terrorism responsibilities of, 72
community: emergency management programs for, 105–6, 108; EOC, equipment issues for, 110; NIMS, importance to, 38–39; NIMS,

# About the Author

Brian J. Gallant has an associate's degree in fire science and safety, a bachelor's degree in management, and a master's degree in education. He spent twelve years in the fire service, serving as training officer, hazardous material officer, department fire investigator, and shift commander (fire lieutenant). Gallant served as an instructor with the Massachusetts Firefighting Academy's Industrial Fire Training Program, specializing in both marine and nuclear firefighting. He was also the Director of Fire Training for Barnstable County, Massachusetts (serving twenty communities on Cape Cod, Massachusetts).

Gallant served as the Emergency Management Director for the Town of Sandwich and, under his regime, handled several major (high-profile) incidents. Among them included two powerful hurricanes, a "no-name" storm, and a barge accident in the Cape Cod Canal area involving hazardous materials and potential evacuation of a large seasonal section of the community.

He was recruited from the fire department to a large nuclear power facility and became a training supervisor, responsible for fire, hazardous materials, safety evaluation, and several other training programs. From the nuclear industry, Gallant went to California to become the regional manager of a full-service environmental consulting firm.

Gallant is currently vice president of Contingency Management Associates, Inc., and is responsible for all environmental, health, and safety training and consulting activities for the Massachusetts-based firm. He has serviced clients worldwide.

He serves as an instructor at Massachusetts Maritime Academy, lecturing in the areas of health and safety, emergency management, OPA 90 training, STCW, marina management, as well as several other courses.

He serves as an associate with a major spill management team. As such, he performs the duties as safety officer at marine and hazardous material related incidents and casualties. Gallant has served as safety/security consultant at several major responses. Additionally, he has trained several marine-related clients and acted as safety officer in drills and exercises.

Gallant is a member of the Barnstable County Deputy Sheriff's Association, the National Association of Fire Investigators, and the American Society of Safety Engineers and is a Certified Hazardous Materials Manager (CHMM).